THE
BACH REMEDIES
REPERTORY

A Supplementary guide
to the use of herbal remedies
discovered by Dr Edward Bach
MB, BS, MRCS, LRCP, DPH

by F. J. Wheeler MRCS, LRCP

Updated, revised and enlarged
by The Dr Edward Bach Centre

SAFFRON WALDEN
THE C.W. DANIEL COMPANY LIMITED

First published in Great Britain 1952
by The C.W. Daniel Company Limited
1 Church Path, Saffron Walden
Essex, CB10 1JP, United Kingdom

First published in 1952 and consequently
reprinted eighteen times
This revised, enlarged and up-dated edition was
published in 1996 and reprinted in 1998 and 2001

ISBN 0 85207 300 3

Produced in association with
Book Production Consultants plc, Cambridge
Typeset by Cambridge Photosetting Services
Printed and bound in England
by St Edmundsbury Press, Bury St Edmunds, Suffolk

PREFACE

Between the years 1930 and 1936 Edward Bach, M.B., B.S., M.R.C.S., L.R.C.P., D.P.H., found, perfected and put into use a system of medicine as simple as it has proved effective. After a successful career in London, he abandoned a lucrative practice to seek and find herbs which would heal the sick, but from which no ill-effects could be derived.

Dr. Bach taught that the basis of disease was to be found in disharmony between the spiritual and mental aspects of a human being. This disharmony, to be found wherever conflicting moods produced unhappiness, mental torture, fear, or lassitude and resignation, lowered the body's vitality and allowed disease to be present. For this reason the remedies he prepared were for the treatment of the mood and temperament of the patient, not for his physical illness; so that each patient becoming more himself could increase his or her own vitality and so draw from an inward strength and an inward peace the means to restore health.

Each patient must lead his own life and learn to lead it in freedom. Each was a different type, a different individual, and each must be treated for his personal mood and the need of the moment, not for his physical disease.

Bach wrote in his book, *The Twelve Healers and Other Remedies*, 'In treating cases with these remedies, no notice is taken of the nature of disease. The individual is treated and as he becomes well the disease goes, having been cast off by the increase in health.

'All know that the same disease may have different effects on different people; it is the effects that need treatment, because they guide to the real cause.

'The mind being the most delicate and sensitive part of the body, shows the onset and the course of disease much more definitely than the body, so that the outlook of mind is chosen as the guide as to which remedy or remedies are necessary.'

Dr. Bach stressed that his remedies could be used in conjunction with any other form of treatment, and would not clash or interfere. Equally, they could achieve great results used alone.

My father, Dr. F. J. Wheeler, who knew and worked with Dr. Bach from 1929 until his death in 1936, and who has himself achieved many remarkable results with the 38 remedies which Dr. Bach produced, set out a repertory for the guidance and help of those who use these remedies.

These indications for the use of the remedies should be studied together with *The Twelve Healers*, to which they are intended to be a supplement. There can be no hard-and-fast rules in treating patients with these remedies, as each patient must be regarded as an individual to be helped in the light of his personal and particular circumstances and moods. But the basic states of mind and the remedies remain constant, and while always bearing in mind the need to retain flexibility and a mind ready to receive fresh inspiration while using these methods of treatment, this repertory should prove of assistance to those seeking to develop their own ability to choose and administer the right remedy either for themselves or for others.

It is in the sincere hope of making yet a further contribution to the understanding of the true art of healing that this book was prepared.

FRANCES M. WHEELER.

London, 1952.

INTRODUCTION TO THE REVISED EDITION

Since this book was first published, it has become a very helpful complement to the more descriptive books on the subject.

The Repertory provides an alphabetical listing of emotions and symptoms, alongside which are suggested remedies relating to the given state of mind. There are many thousands of words to describe the way we feel, and it would be impossible to list every one in a book of this nature. In revising and up-dating *The Bach Remedies Repertory*, it has been our aim to include as many words and cover as many variations as possible, thereby creating a comprehensive index of the most commonly – and in some cases, not so commonly – used terms.

In order to select the most appropriate remedy or remedies, it is important to consider the problem in relation to its cause and how it is experienced on a personal level because the characteristics expressed and experienced by the individual concerned are the guiding factors. For example, listed under DEPRESSION, there are several sub-categories describing a number of different reasons for a depressed state of mind, and the suggested choice of remedy is indicated alongside the most appropriate descriptive term.

Similarly, listed under SENSITIVITY, there are several sub-divisions: *to noise, to controversy, to criticism* and so on, and there are, in turn, a choice of remedies listed within each category. For example, *Sensitivity to noise* suggests Clematis, Mimulus, Water Violet and Impatiens. You would not need all four remedies, but should consider each one separately on its own merits, consulting the descriptive books such as *The Twelve Healers and Other Remedies*, *The Bach Flower Remedies Step by Step*, *The Handbook* or *The Dictionary* for clarification. **Clematis** people are sensitive to noise because they tend to day-dream and therefore find noise disturbs their thoughts. **Mimulus** people tend to be nervous and are therefore frightened by noise. **Water Violet** people enjoy peace and quiet and therefore find noise an intrusion into their privacy. **Impatiens** people think and work quickly, and therefore become irritated by noise because it hinders their progress.

It should be remembered that people interpret words in different ways so there will always be a subjective element to any descriptive term used. The Repertory is intended to be used for clarification when in doubt, to provide a few objective ideas, or simply to jog the memory. Always remember to consider the individual characteristics of the suggestions given because it is only by reading the full description of each remedy before finally deciding upon your choice, that satisfactory results can be obtained.

JUDY HOWARD

Sotwell, 1995   The Dr. Edward Bach Centre

Moods	Remedies
ABANDONED	
fear of being	Mimulus
without hope	Sweet Chestnut
see also REJECTION and LONELINESS	
ABASHED	
with guilt or self-reproach	Pine
ABHORRENCE	
regarding with hatred	Holly
disgust	Crab Apple
ABILITY	
lack of confidence in own	Larch
lack of confidence, momentarily, due to pressure/responsibility	Elm
lack of belief/trust in self	Larch, Cerato
creative (positive)	Clematis
aggressively certain of one's own	Vervain, Vine, Beech, Impatiens
ABNORMALITY	
obsessed with personal defect	Crab Apple
fear of mental	Cherry Plum
thoughts of unfairness – "why me?"	Willow
ABRASIVE	
and critical	Beech, Chicory
and short tempered	Impatiens, Holly
and angry, hateful, jealous, envious	Holly
with resentment, self-pity	Willow, Chicory
and defiant	Vine
ABRUPT	Impatiens, Beech, Vine

Moods	Remedies
ABSENTEEISM	
to avoid responsibilities	Elm
to avoid confrontation	Agrimony
due to lack of interest/escapism	Clematis, Wild Rose, Hornbeam, Mustard
due to fear	Larch, Mimulus, Rock Rose, Rescue Remedy
ABSENT MINDED	
due to drifting thoughts	Clematis
due to tiredness	Olive
ABSORPTION	
with distant thoughts/day-dreaming	Clematis
with memories	Honeysuckle
with enthusiasm or matters of principle	Vervain
with self	Heather, Chicory
with details	Crab Apple
with worries	White Chestnut
with vengeance/jealousy/hatred	Holly
ABSTINENCE	
self-righteous/extreme self control	Rock Water
adjustment to, after e.g. alcoholism	Walnut, Agrimony
ABSTRACT	
ideas and fantasies	Clematis
lacking in ambition	Wild Rose
ABSURDITY	
intolerance with/accusation of	Beech
frustration with	Vervain
ABUSE	
sense of injustice of	Vervain
shock of	Star of Bethlehem
fear of	Mimulus, Rock Rose
sense of contamination by	Crab Apple

Moods	Remedies
ABUSIVE	
due to uncontrolled rage	Cherry Plum
due to aggressive dominance	Vine
due to selfish possessiveness	Chicory
due to vexation	Holly
due to critical intolerance	Beech
due to slowness	Impatiens
due to frustration	Vervain
ACCEPTANCE	
resigned to the inevitable	Wild Rose
meek	Centaury
ACCIDENT PRONE	
due to lack of concentration	Clematis
due to impatience/nervous tension	Impatiens
due to fearful nervousness	Aspen, Mimulus
due to over-enthusiasm	Vervain
ACCOMPLISHMENT	
doubt of one's ability	Larch
eager to achieve	Vervain, Impatiens
ACCUSING	
due to suspicion	Holly
due to desire for perfection	Rock Water, Vervain
as a "put-down"	Beech
due to irrational fears	Cherry Plum
ACHIEVE	
ambitious desire to	Vervain, Vine
doubt of one's ability to	Larch
ACID-TONGUED	
due to spitefulness/hatred	Holly
irritated annoyance/intolerance	Beech
and bitter/selfish	Willow, Chicory
critical, bitingly accusative	Chicory, Beech, Vine
ACQUIESCENCE	
generally	Centaury, Wild Rose
due to fear	Mimulus, Larch

Moods	Remedies
ACQUISITIONS	
desire to cling to, selfishly	Chicory
clings to due to sentimental attachment	Honeysuckle
to aid release of emotional attachment to	Walnut
ACRIMONIOUS	Chicory, Willow, Holly, Vine, Beech
ACTING	
as a pretence	Agrimony
to gain attention/favour	Chicory
ACTIVE	
excessively, due to enthusiasm	Vervain
excessively, due to impatience/ hastiness	Impatiens
overly, as hard task master to self	Rock Water
ADAMANT	Vervain, Vine
ADAPT	
helps to	Walnut
ADAPTABLE	Wild Rose, Clematis
ADDICTION	
life controlled by	Centaury
used as means of escape	Agrimony, Clematis
to break habit of	Walnut, Chestnut Bud
see also WITHDRAWAL	
ADDLED	Scleranthus, Cerato
ADHERENCE	
to principles	Vervain, Rock Water

Moods	Remedies
ADMIRATION	
for others/desire to copy or follow	Cerato
none for self	Pine, Crab Apple
with envy/jealousy	Holly
ADORATION	
for others, with desire to possess	Chicory
of self	Heather, Chicory, Rock Water
none for self	Pine, Crab Apple
ADRENALINE (emotional)	
feeling of having excess	Impatiens, Vervain, Aspen, Rock Rose, Rescue Remedy
ADRIFT	Wild Rose, Clematis
ADULATION	
of self	Heather, Chicory, Rock Water
ADVENTURE	
desire for	Clematis
great spirit of	Vervain
no desire for	Wild Rose, Mustard, Olive
ADVERSITY	
struggles on in spite of	Oak
unaffected by	Oak, Vine, Vervain, Wild Rose
depressed by	Gentian, Gorse
ADVICE	
seeking	Cerato
influenced by and follows	Centaury, Cerato, Walnut
withholds until requested to give	Water Violet
eager to give	Chicory, Vervain
hurt if not taken	Chicory

Moods	Remedies
AFFECTIONATE	Centaury, Chicory, Red Chestnut, Pine
AFRAID	
due to known cause	Mimulus
desperately/panic stricken	Rock Rose, Cherry Plum
irrationally	Cherry Plum, Aspen
due to unknown cause	Aspen
for welfare of others	Red Chestnut
of failure	Larch
see also FEAR	
AFTER-SHOCK	Star of Bethlehem, Rescue Remedy
AGEING	
desire to reverse	Honeysuckle, Heather, Rock Water
dislike of look of self	Crab Apple
fear of	Mimulus, Rock Rose
AGGRAVATING	
due to intensity	Vervain
due to impatience	Impatiens
due to indecision	Scleranthus, Cerato
due to persistence	Vervain, Heather
AGGRAVATED	
by the slowness of others	Impatiens
by the stupidity of others	Beech
by the weakness of others	Vine
by injustice/unfairness	Vervain
AGGRESSION	
enthusiastic/passionate	Vervain
spiteful	Holly
demanding/dominant	Vine

Moods	Remedies
AGGRIEVED	
and resentful	Willow
and hurt	Chicory
and angered by injustice	Vervain
but does not protest	Centaury, Agrimony
AGITATED	Impatiens, Agrimony, White Chestnut
with detail	Crab Apple
with injustice	Vervain
AGONY (emotional)	
concealed, inner torture	Agrimony
of grief	Star of Bethlehem, Sweet Chestnut
of mental arguments	White Chestnut
AGREES	
readily, against better judgement	Cerato, Centaury
to keep peace	Agrimony, Centaury, Wild Rose
AILMENTS	
obsessed with	Crab Apple, Heather
enjoys talking in detail about	Heather
feels unclean due to	Crab Apple
afraid of	Mimulus
exhausted/drained by	Olive
see also ILLNESS	
AIMLESS	Wild Rose, Wild Oat
AIR-HEAD	Clematis

Moods	Remedies
AIR TRAVEL	
fear of	Mimulus, Rock Rose, Rescue Remedy
worried about	White Chestnut, Aspen
exhausted by	Olive
bemused and distracted by	Clematis
adjustment following	Walnut
jet lag	Walnut, Clematis, Olive
AIR-SICK	Rescue Remedy, Scleranthus, Walnut
ALCOHOL	
addiction to	Centaury, Agrimony, Cerato
breaking habit of addiction to	Walnut, Chestnut Bud
sickened by	Crab Apple
repeated hangovers	Chestnut Bud
used as a "crutch", to provide courage	Agrimony, Larch, Mimulus
ALIENATION	
due to aloof distancing	Water Violet
due to over-talkativeness	Heather
due to irritation	Impatiens
due to suffocating possessiveness	Chicory
due to influence/persuasive control of others	Walnut
ALONE	
preference for being	Water Violet
fear of being	Mimulus, Agrimony
dislike of being	Chicory, Heather
to work at own pace	Impatiens
ALOOFNESS	Water Violet
ALTRUISTIC	Oak, Centaury, Red Chestnut, Vervain

Moods	Remedies
AMBITION	
lack of	Wild Rose, Gorse
strong sense of	Vervain, Vine
definite but side-tracked	Walnut
ill-defined	Wild Oat
to possess/control others	Chicory, Vine
delayed/disappointed about, due to set-back	Gentian
AMBIVALENCE	Scleranthus, Cerato
AMUSEMENT	
no sense of	Mustard, Gorse, Willow
malicious/spiteful sense of	Holly, Chicory
pretence – put on "brave/cheerful face"	Agrimony
ANALYTICAL	Rock Water, Beech, Vervain, Vine
ANGER	
due to hatred/envy	Holly
due to injustice	Vervain
uncontrolled	Cherry Plum
with self for weakness	Centaury
with self for hesitancy/indecision	Scleranthus
with self for failure	Rock Water
with slowness	Impatiens
with stupidity of others	Beech
ANGST	Aspen
see also ANXIETY	
ANGUISH	Sweet Chestnut, Agrimony
ANNOYANCE	
with others/trivial matters	Impatiens, Beech
due to physical restrictions of illness	Oak
due to frustration	Vervain, Oak

Moods	Remedies
ANSWER BACK	
for attention	Chicory
resentfully	Willow
spitefully	Holly
with valid argument	Vervain
in defiance	Vine, Vervain, Chicory
ANTICIPATION	
vague fears/foreboding	Aspen
of trouble for others	Red Chestnut
of failure	Larch, Mimulus
ANTI-CLIMAX	Gentian
ANTI-SOCIAL	
appears to be	Water Violet
due to sulkiness	Willow
due to shyness/timidity	Mimulus
due to lack of confidence	Larch
due to self-opinionated/ pretentiousness	Vine
ANXIETY	
hidden/concealed restlessness	Agrimony
known cause	Mimulus
for welfare of others	Red Chestnut
unknown cause/vague anticipation	Aspen
with worrying thoughts	White Chestnut
ANXIOUSNESS	
with vague anticipation	Aspen
for welfare of others	Red Chestnut
concealed, restless	Agrimony
APATHY	
generally	Wild Rose, Hornbeam, Clematis
due to depression	Gorse, Mustard
due to lack of energy/exhaustion	Olive

Moods	Remedies
APOLOGETIC	Pine
APPREHENSIVE	
through fear	Aspen, Mimulus, Rock Rose
for others	Red Chestnut
and doubtful/despondent	Gentian
about possible failure	Larch
APPROVAL	
seeks, for reassurance	Cerato
ARDENT	Vervain
ARGUMENTATIVE	Beech, Vervain, Willow, Chicory, Holly, Impatiens
ARGUMENTS	
mental	White Chestnut
enjoys	Vervain, Chicory, Willow, Beech
avoids	Agrimony, Centaury, Water Violet, Clematis, Wild Rose
ARROGANCE	Beech, Vine
ATTENTION	
seeks	Chicory, Heather, Willow
dislikes	Water Violet
AUTHORITARIAN	Vine
AUTOCRATIC	Vine

Moods	Remedies
AVOIDANCE	
of arguments	Agrimony, Centaury, Water Violet, Clematis, Wild Rose
of people	Water Violet, Mimulus, Beech, Impatiens
of confronting reality	Agrimony, Clematis, Honeysuckle, Chestnut Bud
AWKWARDNESS	
concealed sense of	Agrimony
due to shyness	Mimulus
due to dislike of self	Crab Apple
due to lack of confidence	Larch
due to hesitancy/indecision	Scleranthus
due to apprehension	Aspen
due to subservience; sense of awe	Centaury
in children of feeble/puny build or character	Mimulus, Larch
BABY BLUES	
for no apparent reason	Mustard
with irrational fears/behaviour	Cherry Plum
BACK-CHAT	Beech, Willow, Chicory
BAD NEWS	Star of Bethlehem
BELONGING	
no sense of, due to uncertainty	Cerato, Scleranthus, Larch
no sense of, due to loneliness	Heather, Sweet Chestnut, Mimulus
no sense of, and feels bitter/pities self	Willow, Chicory
no sense of, feels unwanted/ostracised	Willow, Chicory, Mimulus, Crab Apple, Gorse, Sweet Chestnut

Moods	Remedies
BEREAVEMENT	
initial shock/numbness	Star of Bethlehem
dejection, emptiness	Sweet Chestnut
longing for one's own death	Clematis
thoughts filled with past memories	Honeysuckle
for protection and adjustment	Walnut
with sense of guilt/self reproach	Pine
with resentment/self-pity	Willow
BEWILDERED	Clematis
BIG-HEADEDNESS	Vine, Beech
BIGOTRY	Vervain, Vine, Beech, Rock Water
BITCHINESS	Holly, Chicory, Beech
BITTERNESS	Willow, Chicory, Holly
BLABBER	
nervous chatter	Impatiens, Agrimony, Mimulus
for attentive company	Heather, Chicory
obsessive preaching	Vervain
BLAME	
others	Willow, Chicory, Beech, Vine
self	Pine, Crab Apple, Red Chestnut, Centaury, Agrimony
BLASÉ	Wild Rose, Clematis
see also BOREDOM	
BLEMISH	
obsessed with	Crab Apple
BLITHE	Agrimony

Moods	Remedies
BLOCKAGE	
of ability to give love	Chicory, Holly
of progression in life due to frustrated ambition	Walnut, Wild Oat, Gorse, Sweet Chestnut, Willow
due to failure to learn	Chestnut Bud
BLOOD	
fear of	Mimulus, Rock Rose
faints at sight of	Rescue Remedy
revolted by	Crab Apple
BLOODY-MINDED	Beech, Willow, Vine, Chicory, Vervain, Rock Water
BLUNT	
due to intolerance	Beech, Vine
straightforwardness	Water Violet, Rock Water, Oak, Vervain
BLUSHES EASILY	Mimulus, Larch, Pine
see also SELF-CONSCIOUSNESS	
BODY IMAGE	
poor sense of, due to self-dislike	Crab Apple
poor sense of, due to uncertainty	Cerato
poor sense of and tries to hide with joviality	Agrimony
excessively high regard for, imposing strict regime for living	Rock Water
BOISTEROUS	
due to excitement	Impatiens, Vervain
as means of seeking attention/ showing off	Chicory
and disobedient	Vine
purposely, as means of hiding inadequacies	Agrimony

Moods	Remedies
BORE	
talkative	Heather
depressing	Gorse, Willow
BOREDOM	
generally	Clematis, Wild Oat
through impatient expectation	Impatiens
BOSSY	Chicory, Vine, Impatiens, Beech, Vervain
BRAIN-STORM	Cherry Plum
BRAINWASHING	
instrumental in	Vervain, Vine, Chicory, Rock Water
succumb to/influenced by	Walnut, Cerato, Clematis, Wild Rose, Centaury, Agrimony
BRAVE	
by nature	Oak, Vine, Vervain
finds it hard to be, through fear	Mimulus, Aspen, Rock Rose, Agrimony, Centaury
finds it hard to be, through lack of confidence/uncertainty	Larch, Scleranthus, Cerato, Centaury
BREAK-DOWN, mental	
due to over-work/burn-out	Oak, Vervain, Elm, Rock Water
due to mental torment/ restlessness	Agrimony, White Chestnut, Cherry Plum, Impatiens, Scleranthus

Moods	Remedies
BROODY	
about future	Clematis, Gentian
about misfortune	Willow, White Chestnut, Sweet Chestnut
about making decisions	Scleranthus
BUBBLY	Agrimony, Heather, Impatiens, Vervain
BURDEN	
believes one is a burden to others	Pine, Mustard
manipulates attention by claiming one is	Chicory
BURDENED	
with work	Oak, Vervain, Centaury, Rock Water
with responsibility	Elm
with mental torment	White Chestnut, Agrimony
with mental pressure	Elm, White Chestnut, Vervain
BURN-OUT	Olive, Walnut, Oak, Rock Water, Vervain
see also BREAK-DOWN	
CAPABLE	
and reliable	Oak, Water Violet, Vine
but doubtful when under pressure	Elm
but has no confidence	Larch
but easily influenced	Walnut
but fusses	Chicory, Vervain
CAPITULATION	Gorse, Wild Rose, Centaury, Agrimony, Sweet Chestnut

Moods	Remedies
CARELESS	
due to impatience	Impatiens
due to boredom	Clematis
due to tiredness	Olive
CAUTIOUS	
by nature	Oak, Water Violet
due to suspicion	Holly
due to fear	Mimulus, Aspen
due to uncertainty	Scleranthus, Cerato
due to doubt	Cerato, Gentian
CHANGEABLE	Cerato, Scleranthus
CHATTER-BOX	Heather, Agrimony, Cerato, Chicory, Impatiens, Vervain
CHEERFULNESS, false	Agrimony
CLEANSER	Crab Apple
CLOWN	Agrimony
COMMUNICATOR, good	Vervain, Oak, Water Violet
COMPANY	
desires	Agrimony, Chicory, Heather, Cerato, Vervain
aversion to	Impatiens, Mimulus, Water Violet, Larch
COMPETITIVE	Vervain, Vine, Rock Water
COMPLACENCY	Wild Rose, Clematis

Moods	Remedies
COMPLAIN	
about others	Beech, Chicory, Holly, Willow, Impatiens
on principle	Vervain
when ill	Willow, Gorse
never	Centaury, Agrimony, Oak
COMPOSURE	Water Violet, Rock Water, Oak
COMPULSIVE	
habits	Crab Apple
talker	Heather, Chicory, Vervain
eating	Crab Apple, Agrimony
lying, for attention	Heather, Chicory
CONCEALMENT of emotions	Agrimony, Water Violet, Oak
CONCEIT	Beech, Rock Water, Vine, Vervain
CONCENTRATION	
lack of	Clematis, White Chestnut
lack of, through indecision	Scleranthus
lack of, through self-distrust	Cerato
over	Vervain, Rock Water
CONCERNED	
about details	Crab Apple
about others	Chicory, Red Chestnut, Oak, Vervain
about self	Heather, Rock Water, Chicory, Willow
CONDESCENDING	Vine, Water Violet, Rock Water

Moods	Remedies
CONFIDENCE	
lack of	Larch, Cerato, Scleranthus, Elm
CONFIRMATION	
seeks	Cerato
CONFRONTATION	
avoids	Agrimony, Centaury, Clematis, Mimulus
enjoys	Vervain, Vine
CONFUSION	Scleranthus, Cerato, Wild Oat
CONGESTION, mental	
through worry	White Chestnut
through anxiousness for others	Red Chestnut
through selfish absorption	Chicory, Heather
through matters of principle	Vervain
through concern over trivialities	Crab Apple
CONSOLATION	
enjoys and seeks	Willow, Chicory
aversion to	Water Violet
CONSPIRACY	
suspicious of	Holly
irrational fear of	Cherry Plum
CONSTANCY	Walnut
CONTAMINATION	Crab Apple
CONTEMPT	
for others	Beech, Vine, Holly, Impatiens
for self	Crab Apple, Pine
CONTROL	
lack of mental	Cherry Plum
desire to control others	Chicory, Vine

Moods	Remedies
CONVALESCENCE	
fatigue during	Hornbeam, Olive
undefined depression during	Mustard
to assist in adjustment	Walnut
CONVERSATION	
enjoys	Heather, Vervain, Agrimony, Chicory
finds difficult	Mimulus, Larch
finds difficult with mundane/trivial chatter	Water Violet, Impatiens
CONVENTIONS	
fond of	Wild Rose, Rock Water
to break old	Walnut
CONVERT	
desire to	Vervain, Beech, Rock Water
CONVICTION, strong sense of	Vervain, Vine, Rock Water, Chicory
COPE	
copes well, even under pressure	Oak
copes well until under pressure	Elm
COPIES others	Cerato
CORRECT	
wishes to	Chicory, Vervain, Beech
COURAGE	
possesses generally, by nature	Oak
of convictions	Vervain
lack of, due to fear	Mimulus, Aspen, Rock Rose
lack of, due to fear of failure	Larch

Moods	Remedies
COVETOUS	Chicory, Holly
COY	Mimulus
CRAZED	Cherry Plum, Vervain

CRIES EASILY
generally	Chicory, Willow
due to mood changes	Scleranthus
because highly sensitive	Walnut, Mimulus, Centaury
due to indefinable depression/ melancholy	Mustard
due to emotional crisis	Rescue Remedy

see also TEARFULNESS, SENSITIVITY and WEEPINESS

CRITICAL
of others	Beech, Chicory, Vervain
of self	Pine, Rock Water, Crab Apple

CROSS-ROADS of life, uncertainty at	Wild Oat
CRUSADER	Vervain

CURIOSITY
lack of	Wild Rose, Gorse

CYNICISM	Beech, Vine, Holly, Willow, Gorse
DAY-DREAMING	Clematis, Honeysuckle
DAZED	Clematis, Star of Bethlehem

Moods	Remedies
DEATH	
fear of	Mimulus, Rock Rose
desires, with irrational desperation	Cherry Plum
desires, as means of escape	Agrimony, Clematis
morbid obsession with	Clematis, Mustard, Sweet Chestnut
DEBATE	
enjoys	Vervain
DECISION	
unable to make	Scleranthus, Cerato, Wild Oat
good at making	Vervain, Vine, Water Violet
DEFENSIVE	Willow, Holly, Vervain
DEFERENCE	Centaury, Cerato, Agrimony
DEFIANCE	Vine, Beech, Chicory
DEFINITE	
sense of purpose	Walnut, Vervain, Rock Water, Vine
DEJECTION	Sweet Chestnut
DELEGATE	
does so with orders	Vine
finds it hard to; does job oneself	Vervain, Impatiens
too timid to	Mimulus, Centaury
no desire to	Oak, Chicory
happy to be relieved from duty	Wild Rose
feels a failure if has to	Elm, Rock Water
DELIRIUM	Cherry Plum

Moods	Remedies
DELUSIONS	
generally, due to imagination	Aspen, Cherry Plum, Clematis
of grandeur	Cherry Plum, Vervain, Rock Water, Chicory
DEMANDING	Vine, Chicory, Heather
DEMENTED	
with irrational fears/out of control	Cherry Plum
with despair	Sweet Chestnut
with hidden fear/torment	Agrimony
with fear over others	Red Chestnut
with irritation	Impatiens
with confusion/indecision	Scleranthus
DEMONSTRATIVE	
generally	Vervain, Vine, Chicory, Holly, Impatiens
not inclined to be	Agrimony, Centaury, Water Violet
DEMURE	Centaury, Water Violet, Mimulus
DEPENDABLE	Oak
DEPENDENT	
on people to fuss over	Chicory
on people for advice	Cerato
on people to talk to	Heather
on people for support/strength	Centaury
DEPLETED of energy	Olive, Hornbeam, Sweet Chestnut

Moods	Remedies
DEPRESSION	
for known reason; due to set-back	Gentian
cause unknown	Mustard
pessimistic	Gorse, Gentian
hopeless	Gorse
utter dejection	Sweet Chestnut
descends suddenly, like dark cloud	Mustard
introspective	Willow

NB: It is important to treat the cause of the depression e.g. guilt, responsibility etc., as appropriate, in addition to the depression itself.

DESIRE	
lack of	Wild Rose, Olive, Hornbeam
excessive	Impatiens, Vervain, Chicory
denial/suppression of	Agrimony, Water Violet, Rock Water
repulsed by (sexual)	Crab Apple
DESIRABILITY	
no sense of due to poor image of self	Crab Apple
needs reassurance about	Cerato
DESPAIR	
materialistic	Gorse, Gentian
due to terror	Rock Rose
pessimistic hopelessness	Gorse
helpless, heartbroken, utter	Sweet Chestnut
cause unknown	Mustard
through self-blame/guilt	Pine
due to shock	Star of Bethlehem
of living	Cherry Plum
DESPERATION	Cherry Plum, Sweet Chestnut

Moods	Remedies
DESPISE	
others	Holly, Beech
others for slowness	Impatiens
others for weakness	Vine
oneself	Crab Apple, Pine
DESPONDENCY	
through lack of confidence	Larch
from self-reproach/guilt	Pine
through feeling of inadequacy	Elm
from shock, bad news	Star of Bethlehem
through limitation of illness	Oak
from feeling of uncleanliness/ unworthiness	Crab Apple
due to embitterment	Willow
cause unknown	Mustard
through frustration	Vervain
through over-work	Vervain, Oak, Elm
through tiredness	Hornbeam, Olive
through slowness, e.g. of progress	Impatiens
complete anguish	Sweet Chestnut
DESTITUTE	Sweet Chestnut
DESTRUCTIVE	Crab Apple, Holly, Willow, Chicory
DETACHED	Water Violet, Clematis, Impatiens
DETERMINATION	Vervain, Vine, Oak, Rock Water, Impatiens
DEVASTATED	Star of Bethlehem, Sweet Chestnut
DEVIOUS	Holly
DEVOID	Sweet Chestnut, Olive

Moods	Remedies
DEVOUT	Rock Water
DIFFIDENT	Larch, Mimulus, Cerato, Centaury
DIGNITY	Water Violet
DILEMMA	Scleranthus, Wild Oat
DILIGENCE	Vervain, Oak
DIPLOMACY	
lack of	Beech, Impatiens, Vine, Holly, Vervain
DIRECTS	
others in illness etc.	Vine
affairs of others	Chicory, Vine, Vervain
DIRT	
dislike of	Crab Apple
DISAGREE	Vervain, Beech, Rock Water, Vine
DISAPPOINTED	Gentian
DISAPPROVING	Rock Water, Chicory, Beech
DISCIPLINARIAN	Vine
DISCIPLINE, self	Rock Water
DISCONTENTMENT	
with life's ambitions	Wild Oat
with self	Rock Water, Pine, Oak
with others	Willow, Chicory, Beech, Impatiens

Moods	Remedies
DISCOURAGEMENT	Gentian, Elm
DISCUSSION	
enjoys	Vervain
avoids, due to shyness	Mimulus
avoids, due to refusal to confront	Agrimony, Clematis
avoids, due to uncertainty of opinion	Cerato, Scleranthus
DISDAINFUL	
generally	Holly, Beech, Vine
may appear to be	Water Violet, Rock Water, Vervain
of oneself	Larch, Crab Apple, Centaury, Pine
DISGRUNTLED	Willow, Chicory
DISHEARTENED	Gentian
DISINCLINATION	
generally	Wild Rose
due to boredom	Clematis
due to tiredness	Olive, Hornbeam
due to depression	Mustard, Gorse, Willow, Sweet Chestnut
DISLIKE of self	Crab Apple, Pine
DISPASSIONATE	Wild Rose
DISSATISFACTION	
due to unfulfilled ambitions	Wild Oat
due to frustration/restriction	Walnut, Vervain, Impatiens
due to limitations during illness	Oak
from resentment	Willow
from envy, jealousy	Holly
with self	Rock Water, Pine
with others	Beech, Chicory, Vine

Moods	Remedies
DISTANT	Clematis
DISTRACTED	
with thoughts of future	Clematis
with thoughts of past	Honeysuckle
with thoughts of nothing	Clematis
with worries	White Chestnut
by flitting thoughts	Impatiens, Scleranthus
DISTRAUGHT	
with fear and concern for others	Red Chestnut
with events of life	Sweet Chestnut
with irrational fears	Cherry Plum
due to shock/bad news	Star of Bethlehem
DISTRUSTFUL	Holly
DITHER	
due to uncertainty/indecision	Scleranthus, Cerato
due to fear	Mimulus, Rock Rose
DOGMA	
rigidly follows	Rock Water
submits to	Centaury, Wild Rose, Cerato, Mimulus, Larch
rebels against	Vine
DOGMATIC	Vine, Rock Water, Vervain
DOMINATION	Vine, Chicory, Heather, Vervain
DOMINATED	Centaury, Cerato, Mimulus, Agrimony
DOMINEERING	Vine, Chicory
DOUBT	Gentian, Cerato

Moods	Remedies
DOWNCAST	Gentian, Willow, Mustard
DREAD	
apprehensive/terrifying	Aspen, Rock Rose
of known event e.g. performing,	
attending interviews, entertaining	Larch, Mimulus
hidden	Aspen, Agrimony
DREAMS	
night terrors	Aspen, Rock Rose, Rescue Remedy
nightmares	Rock Rose, Star of Bethlehem, Rescue Remedy
recurring	Honeysuckle, Chestnut Bud, Pine, Rescue Remedy
day-dreams	Clematis
vividly imaginative	Clematis, Vervain, Cherry Plum
DRIFTING in life	
due to lack of ambition	Wild Rose
with dissatisfaction due to lack of direction	Wild Oat
DROWSINESS	
dreamy, sleepy	Clematis
due to exhaustion	Olive
due to lethargy/mental weariness	Hornbeam
due to apathy	Wild Rose
DUTIFUL	Centaury
DUTY, great sense of	Rock Water, Oak, Vervain
EAGERNESS	Impatiens, Vervain, Aspen

Moods	Remedies
EATING	
greedily	Impatiens, Vervain
dislike of	Crab Apple
prefers to do so in private	Water Violet
afraid of	Mimulus, Aspen, Rock Rose
EFFICIENT	Oak, Rock Water, Water Violet, Vervain, Vine
EFFORT	
lack of due to dreaminess	Clematis
lack of due to exhaustion	Olive, Hornbeam
lack of due to apathetic resignation	Wild Rose
over	Impatiens, Vervain, Rock Water
EGOTISTIC	Beech, Vine, Vervain
EMBARRASSMENT	Mimulus, Larch, Crab Apple
EMBITTERMENT	Willow
EMERGENCIES	Rescue Remedy
EMOTION	
hides	Agrimony, Water Violet, Oak
flat/apparent absence of	Wild Rose
EMPHATIC	Vervain
ENDURANCE	Oak, Centaury, Vervain, Rock Water

Moods	Remedies
EMPTY	
due to exhaustion	Olive
due to lack of interest	Clematis, Honeysuckle
due to sorrow	Star of Bethlehem
due to utter dejection	Sweet Chestnut
ENERGY	
lack of	Olive, Hornbeam, Wild Rose
excess of	Impatiens, Vervain, Aspen
ENMITY	Holly
ENRAGED	
generally	Holly, Cherry Plum
about injustice	Vervain
ENTHUSIASTIC	Vervain
ENVY	Holly
EQUITY, great belief in	Vervain
ESCAPISM, mental	Clematis, Honeysuckle, Agrimony
EXACTITUDE	Rock Water, Vervain, Beech
EXAMINATIONS	
nervousness prior to	Mimulus, Rescue Remedy, Aspen, Larch
lethargy prior to	Hornbeam
exhaustion due to	Olive
despondent over	Gentian
indifference/lack of concentration	Wild Rose, Clematis

Moods	Remedies
EXAMPLE	
would like to be, for others to follow	Rock Water
EXAGGERATES	
due to enthusiasm	Vervain
due to imagination	Clematis, Cherry Plum
for sympathy and attention	Chicory, Heather
of symptoms	Heather
EXASPERATION	Vervain, Beech, Impatiens, Sweet Chestnut
EXCESSIVE	Agrimony, Vervain, Impatiens, Cherry Plum, Crab Apple
EXCITABLE	Impatiens, Vervain, Heather, Agrimony
EXCITEMENT	
seeks, desires, anxious for	Clematis, Agrimony, Heather
lacks emotional	Wild Rose, Hornbeam, Gorse, Mustard
unexplained feeling of	Aspen, Impatiens, Vervain
EXHAUSTION	
through overwork, due to weak will	Centaury
physical and mental	Olive
mental weariness/procrastination	Hornbeam
through strain and effort	Vervain
through lack of vitality	Clematis, Wild Rose
struggles on in spite of	Oak
with extreme helplessness/despair	Sweet Chestnut

Moods	Remedies
EXPECTANT	Aspen, Impatiens
EXPERIENCE	
does not learn from	Chestnut Bud
EXPRESSION	
lacks	Wild Rose
avoids	Agrimony, Water Violet
glum	Mustard, Gorse, Willow
EXTROVERT	
by nature	Vervain, Vine, Impatiens, Heather
as a mask	Agrimony
EYE-CONTACT	
avoids nervously	Mimulus, Aspen
avoids due to embarrassment	Mimulus, Larch, Pine, Crab Apple
avoids due to shyness/timidity	Mimulus, Centaury
avoids to hide feelings	Agrimony
powerful, intense	Vervain, Vine, Chicory, Heather, Impatiens
intense, but agitated due to nervous energy	Impatiens
stares dreamily/looks through subject	Clematis
close to face, direct	Heather
FABRICATION	
to get attention	Heather, Chicory, Willow
due to over-active imagination	Clematis, Cherry Plum
malicious	Holly
FACADE	Agrimony

Moods	Remedies
FAILURE	
expects/fears	Larch, Mimulus
temporary feeling of	Elm
to reach high standards	Rock Water
to others	Pine
FAINTNESS	Clematis
FAIRNESS	
great belief in	Vervain
FAITH	
lost	Gentian, Gorse, Sweet Chestnut
lacks in oneself	Cerato, Elm, Larch
FAMILY	
over-concerned with	Chicory, Red Chestnut
FANATICAL	Vervain
FANTASIES	Clematis, Cherry Plum
FAULT-FINDING	
with others	Beech, Chicory, Holly, Impatiens, Willow, Vervain
with self	Pine, Rock Water, Crab Apple

Moods	Remedies
FEAR	
known cause (illness, poverty, pain etc.)	Mimulus
unknown cause	Aspen
of darkness	Aspen, Mimulus
of death	Aspen, Mimulus, Rock Rose
of fear	Aspen
extreme	Rock Rose
of insanity	Cherry Plum
of failure	Larch
of future	Aspen, Mimulus, Agrimony
for oneself when ill/for one's health	Heather, Mimulus
of losing friends	Chicory, Heather, Mimulus
of mind giving way/loss of control	Cherry Plum
of God	Aspen, Mimulus
secret	Aspen, Mimulus, Agrimony, Scleranthus
vague, unreasoning	Aspen
for oneself if ill	Heather, Mimulus
absence of, for self	Red Chestnut
FEARFUL, by nature	Mimulus
FEARLESS	Oak
FERVENCY	Vervain
FICKLE	Scleranthus, Cerato
FIERY	Holly, Vervain, Impatiens, Cherry Plum
FIGHTING SPIRIT	Vervain, Oak

Moods	Remedies
FIXATION	
with project	Vervain
with injustice	Vervain
with self	Heather, Crab Apple
with detail	Crab Apple
with cleanliness	Crab Apple
FIXED IDEAS & OPINIONS	Beech, Rock Water, Vervain, Vine
FLIPPANT	Impatiens, Holly
FLOATING, sensation of	Clematis
FOLLOWS others	
due to uncertainty	Cerato
because eager to please	Centaury
due to lack of self-confidence	Larch
FOOLISH	Cerato
FORCEFUL	Vine
FREEDOM	
yearning desire for (from torment)	Sweet Chestnut, Clematis, Agrimony, Cherry Plum
desires, from responsibility	Elm
desires, from duty	Centaury
feels claustrophobic without	Water Violet, Impatiens
FORGETFUL	
due to mental turmoil	White Chestnut, Agrimony
due to lack of concentration	Clematis
due to apathy	Wild Rose
FORGIVE	
unable to, due to bitterness	Willow
unable to, due to injustice	Vervain
readily does so, as blames self	Pine, Centaury

Moods	Remedies
FORTITUDE	Oak
FRANTIC	
with worry	White Chestnut
with worry/anxiety over others	Red Chestnut
with irrational fears	Cherry Plum, Aspen
in crisis situation	Rescue Remedy
FRETFUL	Chicory, Agrimony, White Chestnut, Red Chestnut
FRIGHT	Star of Bethlehem, Rock Rose
FRUSTRATION	
generally	Vervain, Walnut
with slowness	Impatiens
uncontrollable	Cherry Plum
FULFILMENT	
lack of, thus seeks	Wild Oat
FUSSINESS	
over other people's affairs/ meddling	Chicory
over others, due to fear/anxiety	Red Chestnut
about detail, trivialities and cleanliness	Crab Apple
about making judgement	Cerato
about principles	Vervain
about correctness	Rock Water, Vervain
FUTURE	
fear of	Aspen, Mimulus, Agrimony
looks forward to	Clematis
has no interest in	Honeysuckle
worries about	White Chestnut, Agrimony

Moods	Remedies
GABBLE	Heather, Impatiens, Agrimony, Vervain
GAIETY, false	Agrimony
GARRULOUS	Heather, Impatiens, Agrimony, Vervain
GAWKISH	Mimulus, Clematis
GENIAL, joyous	Agrimony
GIGGLE	
to hide feelings	Agrimony
nervously	Mimulus, Agrimony, Larch
with nervous impatience	Impatiens
GLOOM	Gorse, Mustard, Willow
GOD	
fear of	Mimulus, Aspen
fear of due to guilt	Pine
self-righteous fear of	Rock Water, Crab Apple
disbelief in	Gorse
anger/hatred of	Holly
bitterness/resentment of	Willow
loss of faith in	Sweet Chestnut
GREEDY	
for others' possessions	Chicory
for sympathy	Chicory, Heather, Willow
for information/advice	Cerato
for power/control	Vine, Chicory, Vervain
for perfection	Rock Water, Vervain
for love	Chicory
for company	Heather

Moods	Remedies
GREGARIOUS	Agrimony, Heather
GRIEF	
sudden, shock	Star of Bethlehem, Rescue Remedy
grieves silently	Water Violet
chronic grieving despair	Sweet Chestnut
heartache	Sweet Chestnut, Star of Bethlehem
with longing for the past	Honeysuckle
with guilt/self blame	Pine
with self condemnation/disgust	Crab Apple
GRIEVANCE	
voices	Vervain, Holly, Vine
does not complain	Centaury, Agrimony, Mimulus, Larch
allows to fester inwardly	Willow, Chicory, White Chestnut, Holly, Agrimony
GRUDGE, bearing	Willow, Chicory
GRUMBLE	Willow
GUIDANCE	
seeks	Cerato
gives	Vervain, Vine, Chicory
gives through criticism	Beech
gives by example	Rock Water
gives quietly when asked	Water Violet
GUILT	Pine
GULLIBLE	Cerato, Clematis
HABITS	
irritated by	Beech
to break	Walnut, Chestnut Bud

Moods	Remedies
HALLUCINATE	Cherry Plum, Rock Rose, Clematis, Vervain, Agrimony
HAND-WASHING	
obsessive, due to sense of uncleanliness	Crab Apple
see also DIRT	
HAPPY-GO-LUCKY	Agrimony, Oak
HAPPINESS	
longs for	Clematis, Star of Bethlehem, Sweet Chestnut
HAPPEN	
fears something is about to	Aspen
can't wait for things to	Impatiens, Clematis
HARD TASK-MASTERS	
to themselves	Rock Water
to others	Beech, Chicory, Vine, Impatiens
HARRASSED	
sense of being/irritated by	Impatiens, Vervain, Cherry Plum
sense of being, due to responsibility	Elm, White Chestnut
and bad-tempered	Impatiens, Vervain, Cherry Plum, Holly, Willow, Beech
ever willing but over-burdened	Centaury, White Chestnut
HASTY	Impatiens

Moods	Remedies
HATE	
generally	Holly
festering resentment	Willow
can see no redeeming features in others	Beech
HAUGHTY	
appears to be, through pride/dignity	Water Violet
if self-opinionated/know-all/autocratic	Vine
through vanity/self obsessed	Heather
through self-righteousness	Rock Water
HAUNTING THOUGHTS	
suffers	Aspen, White Chestnut, Honeysuckle
protection from	Walnut
HEADSTRONG	Vervain, Vine
HELP	
in emergencies/distress	Rescue Remedy
seeks help in decision making	Cerato
HELPFUL	
but maintains discreet distance	Water Violet
calmly, without question	Oak
but fusses	Chicory, Vervain
dutifully, eager to please	Centaury, Pine
HELPLESSNESS	Sweet Chestnut
HESITANCY	
through uncertainty	Scleranthus, Cerato
through fear	Mimulus
through lack of confidence	Larch
none, being self-assured	Impatiens, Vine, Water Violet, Vervain, Chicory

Moods	Remedies
HIGHLY STRUNG	Vervain, Rock Water, Impatiens
through anticipation/living on a knife-edge	Aspen
HOME-SICKNESS	Honeysuckle
HOPELESSNESS	
pessimistic	Gorse
extreme	Sweet Chestnut
HORRIFIED	Rock Rose, Star of Bethlehem
HOSTILITY	
due to hatred/suspicion/envy/ jealousy	Holly
due to intolerance	Beech
due to irritation with slowness	Impatiens
HOUSE-PROUD	Crab Apple, Chicory, Rock Water
HUMOUR	
hides emotions behind, like clown	Agrimony
lacks sense of	Willow, Mustard, Gorse
HYGIENE	
obsessed with	Crab Apple
HYPERACTIVE	Vervain, Impatiens, Cherry Plum
HYPNOTISED	Clematis
HYPOCHONDRIA	Heather, Crab Apple
HYPOCRISY	Scleranthus, Cerato, Centaury, Agrimony

Moods	Remedies
HYSTERIA	Cherry Plum, Rescue Remedy
IDEALISTIC	
of future/fantasies	Clematis
impractically	Clematis
over-enthusiastic perfectionism	Vervain
for self	Rock Water
high ideals	Vervain, Beech, Impatiens, Rock Water
unable to realise ambitions	Wild Oat
IDENTITY	
lack of	Cerato, Agrimony, Centaury
ILLNESS	
simulated	Chicory, Heather, Willow
frustrated by	Oak
feels unclean during	Crab Apple
fear of	Mimulus
depleted energy due to/help in convalescence	Olive
see also AILMENTS	
IMAGE	
lacks definition	Cerato, Centaury
dislikes one's own	Crab Apple, Pine
high opinion of one's own	Rock Water, Heather, Chicory, Vine
IMAGINATION	
creative	Clematis
over-zealous	Cherry Plum, Rock Rose
lacks	Wild Rose, Gorse
vivid	Clematis, Cherry Plum
influenced by	Walnut

Moods	Remedies
IMITATES	
through lack of self-identity/ certainty	Cerato
because easily led	Centaury, Walnut
IMMEDIACY	
demands	Impatiens, Vine
IMPARTIALITY	Wild Rose, Scleranthus, Cerato, Clematis
IMPATIENT	Impatiens
IMPETUOUS	Impatiens, Vervain, Cherry Plum
IMPRESSION	
tries to make	Willow, Chicory
tries to make, for sympathy	Willow, Chicory
tries to make, in order to convert	Vervain
tries to make, as example	Rock Water
IMPUDENT	Willow, Chicory, Beech
IMPULSIVE	
quick and eager/hasty/impetuous	Impatiens
irrational/uncontrolled/fear of	Cherry Plum
over-enthusiastic/hasty	Vervain
acts out imaginary fantasy	Clematis
becoming a salve to impulses	Centaury, Walnut
IMPURITY	
dislikes/feels contaminated by	Crab Apple
INADEQUACY	
through lack of confidence	Larch, Elm
through self-distrust	Cerato, Scleranthus
through guilt	Pine
through fear/shyness/timidity	Mimulus

Moods	Remedies
INATTENTIVE	Clematis, Honeysuckle, White Chestnut
INCENSED	Vervain
INDECISION	Scleranthus
about life's direction	Wild Oat
about one's judgement/instincts	Cerato
INDEPENDENCE	Water Violet, Oak Impatiens, Vine
INDIFFERENCE	
to life	Clematis, Wild Rose, Mustard
towards needs of others	Beech, Vine, Chicory, Holly, Impatiens
INDIGNANT	Chicory, Vervain, Beech
INDULGENCE	
in food, then feels disgusted	Crab Apple
in projects, enthusiastically	Vervain
hurriedly	Impatiens
refrains from, through politeness	Water Violet
refrains from, through self-restraint	Rock Water
needs protection from	Walnut
INERTIA	Hornbeam, Wild Rose
through exhaustion	Olive
through depression	Mustard, Gorse
INFURIATED	Holly, Vervain, Vine Cherry Plum, Beech

Moods	Remedies
INFLUENCED	
from path in life	Walnut, Cerato, Wild Oat
easily, by dominance of others	Centaury
by decision of others	Cerato, Gorse, Centaury, Agrimony
by delay and hindrance	Gentian
for the sake of peace	Agrimony
through jealousy/envy	Holly
INQUISITIVE	Vervain, Impatiens, Chicory, Clematis
INSANITY	
fears	Cherry Plum
sense of	Clematis
sense of, due to frustration	Vervain, Impatiens
INSECURITY	
generally	Cerato, Larch
through fear	Mimulus, Red Chestnut
and clings to others	Heather, Chicory
needs to be loved/protected	Chicory
INSENSITIVE	Vine, Beech, Chicory
INSTANT	
desires instant action	Impatiens, Vervain
INSTINCTS	
follows	Vervain
distrusts	Cerato, Scleranthus
INTENSE	Vervain

Moods	Remedies
INTEREST	
lack of, due to distant thoughts	Clematis, Honeysuckle
lack of, due to fatigue	Olive, Hornbeam
lack of, due to apathy/resignation	Wild Rose
lack of, due to worry	White Chestnut
lack of, due to depression	Gorse, Mustard
lack of, due to self-absorption	Heather
lack of, through embitterment	Willow
too much, generally, especially matters of principle	Vervain
too much, in affairs of others	Chicory
INTERFERENCE	
in affairs of others	Chicory
by fussing and criticising	Chicory
by talking of self	Heather
by dominating	Vine
by persuasion	Vervain
by asking questions	Cerato
by revenge	Holly
by thoughts/mental arguments	White Chestnut
by setting rigid example	Rock Water
no desire for	Water Violet
protection from	Walnut
INTERVIEW	
nervousness about	Rescue Remedy, Mimulus, Larch
negative about	Gentian, Gorse
fearful/worried about	Mimulus, White Chestnut
INTIMIDATED	Centaury, Mimulus, Walnut, Agrimony
INTIMIDATING	Vine
INTOLERANCE	Beech
of slowness	Impatiens
of inaccuracy	Vervain, Rock Water

Moods	Remedies
INTROSPECTION	Willow, Heather
through guilt	Pine
INTROVERTED	Centaury, Mimulus
due to dreaminess	Clematis
due to sulkiness/self-pity	Willow
appears to be, due to dignified aloofness	Water Violet
through worry	White Chestnut
through indecision	Scleranthus
for selfish reasons	Chicory
INTUITION, distrusts	Cerato
INVOKES ILLNESS	
to obtain sympathy	Chicory, Heather
to manipulate others	Chicory
through resentment/self-pity	Willow
to escape from reality	Clematis
to escape fear	Mimulus
due to lack of confidence	Larch
IRRATIONAL	
thoughts generally	Cherry Plum
fears of harmful act	Cherry Plum
anxiety	Aspen
IRRITABILITY	
generally	Impatiens
with mannerisms and habits of others	Beech
due to selfishness	Chicory
due to ill temper	Holly, Willow
due to frustration with insensitivity/injustices	Vervain
ISOLATION	
enjoys	Water Violet, Impatiens
cannot bear	Heather

Moods	Remedies
JADED	Olive, Hornbeam
JEALOUSY	Holly
JOKES	
to make light of problems	Agrimony
JOVIALITY, false	Agrimony
JUDGEMENTS	
distrusts one's own	Cerato
suspicious/distrustful of others'	Holly
afraid of	Mimulus, Rock Rose
makes hasty	Impatiens
overly critical	Vervain, Beech
JUMPY	Mimulus, Impatiens, Aspen, Agrimony
JUSTICE	
great belief in	Vervain
KARMA	
submission to	Clematis
unquestioned acceptance of	Wild Rose
afraid of consequences of	Mimulus, Aspen, Rock Rose
over influenced by/feels controlled	Walnut, Crab Apple, Centaury
KEEN	Vervain
KEEPSAKES	
sentimental about	Honeysuckle
no attachment to	Clematis
irritated by	Impatiens, Beech, Vine
comforted by	Centaury, Mimulus, Larch, Cerato, Honeysuckle, Chicory

Moods	Remedies
KILL	
irrational desire to	Cherry Plum
hateful desire to	Holly
over-concerned about accidental killing of insects	Red Chestnut, Pine, Centaury
over-concerned about slaughter of animals	Red Chestnut, Vervain, Centaury, Pine
KNOW-ALL	Vine, Beech
KNOWS BEST	Chicory, Vervain, Rock Water, Water Violet
LABORIOUS, work seems	Hornbeam, Wild Rose
LASSITUDE	
generally	Hornbeam, Wild Rose, Olive, Clematis
due to self-pity/resentment	Willow
due to depression	Gorse, Mustard, Sweet Chestnut
LAUGHTER	
to hide feelings	Agrimony
nervous	Agrimony, Impatiens, Mimulus
uncontrollable	Cherry Plum
LAX	Wild Rose, Clematis, Hornbeam, Scleranthus, Cerato, Larch
LAZINESS	Wild Rose, Hornbeam, Clematis

Moods	Remedies
LEADERSHIP	Vine, Vervain, Water Violet
LEARN	
unable to, from experience/ mistakes	Chestnut Bud
LECTURE	
desire to, due to enthusiasm	Vervain
does so, to dominate/control	Vine
does so, to get own way	Chicory
does so, to expose stupidity	Beech
LETHARGY	
generally	Hornbeam, Wild Rose
despises	Rock Water
LIBERATION	
desire for	Sweet Chestnut, Clematis, Cherry Plum
desire for, from duty	Centaury
desire for, from mental torment	White Chestnut, Agrimony
LIFE	
despaired of	Sweet Chestnut, Rescue Remedy
seems a drudgery	Centaury, Hornbeam, Olive, Gorse
loss of interest in	Clematis, Gorse
no pleasure in	Olive, Mustard
irrational desire to end	Cherry Plum
LIVELY	Impatiens, Vervain, Agrimony
LIVID	Holly, Vervain, Cherry Plum, Vine

Moods	Remedies
LOATHSOME	
of others	Holly
of self	Crab Apple
LONELINESS	
enjoys	Water Violet
prefers, for work	Impatiens
dislikes	Agrimony, Heather, Chicory, Mimulus, Vervain
seeks, as an escape	Clematis
heartbreaking	Star of Bethlehem, Sweet Chestnut
LONGS FOR	
peace of mind	White Chestnut, Agrimony
home	Honeysuckle
loved ones	Honeysuckle, Chicory, Red Chestnut
freedom from mental torture	Agrimony, White Chestnut, Scleranthus, Sweet Chestnut, Cherry Plum
future, for better times	Clematis
something to look forward to	Clematis
release from envy, jealousy	Holly
LOSS	
sense of, e.g. through grief	Star of Bethlehem
see also BEREAVEMENT and GRIEF	
LOVE	
lack of, for others	Holly
lack of, for self	Crab Apple, Pine
desires more of/constant	Chicory
desires as reassurance	Cerato

Moods	Remedies
LOVE-STRUCK	
and dreamy	Clematis
but jealous	Holly
but possessive/clinging	Chicory
LOW	
in spirits	Mustard, Olive, Sweet Chestnut, Gentian, Gorse, Willow
see also DEPRESSION and DOWNCAST	
LUNACY	Cherry Plum, Agrimony, Impatiens
LUST	Chicory, Vervain, Heather, Cherry Plum
MACABRE thoughts	Mustard, Cherry Plum, White Chestnut
MADNESS	Cherry Plum
MADDENING	
finds subject matter	Vervain
finds people	Vervain, Beech, Vine
finds slowness	Impatiens
MALICIOUS	
tendencies	Holly
thoughts, mental arguments	White Chestnut, Holly, Willow
MALINGER	
due to responsibility	Elm
due to exhaustion	Olive
due to laziness	Wild Rose

Moods	Remedies
MANIC	
thoughts	Cherry Plum, White Chestnut
with depression	Mustard, Scleranthus
suicidal	Cherry Plum
MANIPULATIVE	Chicory
MANIPULATED	Centaury, Agrimony
MANNERISMS	
irritated by	Beech
irritated by slowness of	Impatiens
uses plentifully to illustrate point	Vervain
MARTYR	
to a cause	Vervain
for affection/attention	Chicory, Heather
to resentment	Willow
to own ideals	Rock Water
as an example to others	Rock Water
MASK	
jovial, to hide fears, worries etc.	Agrimony
MASOCHISM, mental	Rock Water, Crab Apple, Pine, Cherry Plum, White Chestnut
MASQUERADE	Agrimony
MASTERFUL	Vervain, Vine
MAZE	
as though lost in	Wild Oat, Scleranthus, Clematis
MEDDLE	
to control/manipulate	Chicory
to hasten	Impatiens
to convince	Vervain

Moods	Remedies
MEDITATIVE	Clematis
MEEK	Centaury, Mimulus, Larch
MEGALOMANIA	Cherry Plum, Vervain, Rock Water, Chicory
MELANCHOLIA	Gorse, Sweet Chestnut
with no known reason	Mustard
MEMORY	
bad, due to lack of concentration	Clematis, Honeysuckle
bad, due to mind full of other things	Vervain, White Chestnut
MENTAL ARGUMENTS	White Chestnut
MERCILESS	Vine, Holly
MERRIMENT	
which hides true feelings	Agrimony
METABOLISM (of mental energy)	
lethargic	Hornbeam, Wild Rose
hyperactive	Impatiens, Vervain
hyperactive, due to fear/anxiety	Rock Rose, Aspen
slow, dreamy	Clematis
slow, through depression	Mustard, Gorse, Sweet Chestnut
METAMORPHOSIS	
helps during	Walnut
METHODICAL	Oak, Rock Water, Vervain, Wild Rose

Moods	Remedies
METICULOUS	
generally, by nature	Rock Water, Vervain, Beech
over concentration to detail	Crab Apple
MIMIC	
due to uncertainty about self	Cerato
sarcastically/spitefully/to gain advantage	Holly, Willow, Chicory
MISANTHROPY	Holly, Beech
MISBEHAVIOUR	
to gain attention	Chicory, Heather, Willow
due to strength of own will	Vine
due to desire for own way	Vine, Chicory
due to fear	Mimulus, Rock Rose
due to being misled by stronger personality	Centaury, Walnut
in trying to impress	Agrimony, Chicory
due to being misled by stronger personalities	Centaury, Cerato, Walnut
MISERY	
generally, in outlook	Willow
with self pity	Willow, Chicory
with pessimism/doubt	Gentian, Gorse
with cloud of depression	Mustard
with bleak despair	Sweet Chestnut
hidden	Agrimony, Water Violet, Oak, Centaury
MISGUIDED BY OTHERS	Centaury, Cerato
on occasions	Walnut
MISTAKES	
does not learn by	Chestnut Bud
blames self for mistakes of others	Pine

Moods	Remedies
MISTRUSTFUL	
of others	Holly
of self	Cerato
of self to do harm/act irrationally	Cherry Plum
MOAN	Willow, Chicory, Gorse
MOCK	Holly, Vine, Beech
MODEST	Centaury, Larch, Mimulus
MONOTONE	Mustard, Gorse, Wild Rose
MOODY	
depression comes and goes	Mustard
mood swings	Scleranthus
self-pitying, selfish	Willow, Chicory
MOPE	Willow, Chicory, Mustard, Gorse
MORALITY	
for self perfectionism	Rock Water
in support of others	Vervain
MORBID THOUGHTS	Mustard, Cherry Plum, White Chestnut
MOTHERLY	Chicory
possessively/selfishly/fussily	Chicory
selflessly anxious	Red Chestnut
gentle and selflessly protective	Centaury
MOTIVATION	
high degree of	Vervain, Vine, Impatiens
lack of, through listlessness	Wild Rose, Hornbeam, Olive

Moods	Remedies
MOULDING OF CHARACTER	
those who try to convert others	Vervain, Chicory, Rock Water
those who are affected by others	Cerato, Walnut, Centaury, Agrimony
MOURNING	
in grief	Star of Bethlehem
with memories/regrets	Honeysuckle
with bleak despair	Sweet Chestnut
with self-reproach/regrets	Pine
and desiring own demise	Clematis
NAG	Chicory, Beech, Vine
NARROW-MINDED	Rock Water, Beech
NAUSEOUS	
feeling of, generally	Crab Apple
with fear	Mimulus, Rock Rose
due to travel	Scleranthus
NERVOUS BREAKDOWN	Cherry Plum, Oak, Scleranthus, Vervain, Agrimony, White Chestnut
NERVOUSNESS	
generally, fearful/timid/shy	Mimulus
with vague anticipation	Aspen
with impatient eagerness	Impatiens
NERVY	Agrimony, Chicory, Impatiens, Mimulus, Vervain
NEUROSIS	Cherry Plum, Rock Rose

Moods	Remedies
NOISE	
aversion to/peace disturbed by	Water Violet, Clematis, Mimulus, Walnut
intolerant of/annoyed with	Beech, Impatiens, Willow
NOSEY	Chicory, Heather, Vervain, Cerato
NOSTALGIA	Honeysuckle
NUISANCE	
apologises for being	Pine
annoyed with/irritated by	Beech, Impatiens
NUMBNESS	Clematis, Star of Bethlehem
OBEDIENCE	
demands	Vine
demands of self	Rock Water
OBEDIENT	Centaury, Cerato, Agrimony
through fear	Mimulus
OBESITY	
disgusted by	Crab Apple
due to over indulgence, acting as crutch	Walnut, Centaury, Wild Rose, Gorse
see also EATING	
OBLIGATION	
feels under, due to sense of duty	Centaury, Pine
feels under, due to sense of principle	Vervain, Oak

Moods	Remedies
OBLIVION	
desires	Clematis, Sweet Chestnut
OBSERVATION	
astute	Impatiens, Vervain, Rock Water
lack of	Clematis, Chestnut Bud, Honeysuckle, White Chestnut, Wild Rose
OBSESSIVE	
fear	Cherry Plum, Rock Rose
religiously	Rock Water, Vervain
with self-righteousness	Rock Water, Chicory
over details	Crab Apple
OBSTINATE	Vervain, Vine, Beech
OBSTRUCTIVE	Beech, Vervain, Vine, Willow, Holly,
OFFENSE	
takes easily with introspection	Chicory, Willow
takes easily due to uncertainty	Cerato, Larch
takes easily due to injustice	Vervain
OLD TIES, TO BREAK	Walnut
OMNIPOTENT	Vine
OPINIONATED	Vine, Vervain, Beech, Chicory, Impatiens

Moods	Remedies
OPPORTUNITY	
loses through doubt	Cerato, Gentian
loses through lack of confidence	Larch
loses through indecision	Scleranthus
loses through lack of faith in intuition	Cerato
loses through uncertainty of vocational path	Wild Oat
OPTIONS	
undecided when confronted with	Scleranthus
confused about ambitions	Wild Oat
doubtful of own mind	Cerato, Scleranthus
OSTENTATION	Beech, Chicory, Heather, Vine
OSTRASISED	
due to selfishness/possessiveness	Chicory
due to unrelenting talkativeness	Heather
due to angry attitude	Holly, Willow
due to critical attitude	Beech, Chicory
OUTBURST	
uncontrolled	Cherry Plum
angered by injustice	Vervain
of hateful/spiteful abuse	Holly
OUTRAGE	
deep sense of	Vervain
OVERACT	
for sympathy or attention	Chicory, Willow

Moods	Remedies
OVER-ANXIOUS	
to please	Centaury
to care for others	Chicory
to influence others	Vervain
for others' opinions	Cerato
over details	Crab Apple
for self	Heather, Rock Water, Willow
for safety of others	Red Chestnut
to set good example	Rock Water
OVER-INDULGENCE	
generally	Vervain, Heather, Chicory
and feels disgusted	Crab Apple
uncontrolled	Cherry Plum
help in breaking habit of	Walnut, Chestnut Bud
OVERRULES	Vine
OVER-SENSITIVITY	
hides	Agrimony
through weakness	Centaury
to strong influences	Walnut
to fancied insults/suspicion	Holly, Vervain
OVERWHELMED	
by responsibility/pressure	Elm
by demands of others	Centaury, Mimulus
harrassed/irritated with constant demands	Impatiens
OVERWORK	
tendency to	Oak, Vervain, Centaury
exhausted by	Olive

Moods	Remedies
OVERWROUGHT	
with fear for others	Red Chestnut
with despair	Sweet Chestnut
with anxiety about how to cope	Elm
with anxiety and foreboding	Aspen
with worry	White Chestnut
PACIFIST	Agrimony, Centaury, Vervain, Clematis, Wild Rose, Oak
PANGS OF GUILT	Pine
PANIC	
generally	Rock Rose, Rescue Remedy
with irrational thoughts	Cherry Plum
PARANOIA	
with suspicion	Holly
with irrational fears	Cherry Plum
PARTICULAR	
over detail	Crab Apple, Rock Water
about self-perfection	Rock Water
about cleanliness	Crab Apple
about upholding principles	Vervain
PASSIONATE	
with enthusiasm	Vervain, Impatiens
without control	Cherry Plum
PASSIVE	Centaury, Mimulus, Wild Rose, Clematis

Moods	Remedies
PAST	
nostalgic memories of	Honeysuckle
no interest in	Clematis
regrets	Honeysuckle, Pine, Crab Apple
to let go of	Walnut
PATH IN LIFE	
to help determine	Wild Oat
to help remain upon	Walnut
PATRONISING/condescending	Vine, Beech, Rock Water
PEACE OF MIND	
disturbed by thoughts/worry	White Chestnut, Agrimony
disturbed by guilt	Pine
disturbed by mental arguments	White Chestnut, Vervain
disturbed by fear	Mimulus, Aspen, Rock Rose
disturbed by fear for others	Red Chestnut
disturbed by grief	Star of Bethlehem, Honeysuckle
disturbed by resentment	Willow
disturbed by indecision	Scleranthus
disturbed by obsession	Crab Apple
PEACE AND QUIET	
enjoys, must have	Water Violet
avoids	Agrimony, Heather
PEEVED	Impatiens, Beech, Vervain
PENSIVE	Clematis
PERFECTIONISM	Beech, Rock Water, Vervain, Vine

Moods	Remedies
PERSECUTION	
suspicious of	Holly, Cherry Plum
afraid of	Cherry Plum, Mimulus, Aspen
PERSISTENT	Vervain, Oak, Rock Water
PERSUASIVE	
enthusiastically	Vervain
quietly	Water Violet
PERSUADED BY OTHERS	
against inclination	Gorse, Wild Rose, Walnut
through self-distrust	Cerato
through weakness	Centaury
through kindness	Agrimony
through jealousy, envy	Holly
to please others	Centaury
PESSIMISM	Gorse, Gentian
PETRIFIED	Rock Rose
PETTY	Crab Apple, Chicory, Beech
PETULANT	Impatiens, Willow
PHILOSOPHICAL	
generally, by nature	Oak, Water Violet, Clematis, Wild Rose
with strong opinions	Vervain
PHOBIAS	
known, generally	Mimulus, Rock Rose, White Chestnut
about dirt/contamination/looks	Crab Apple
unknown/vague	Aspen
irrational	Cherry Plum

Moods	Remedies
PIOUS	Rock Water, Beech
PINE	Honeysuckle, Clematis
PITY	
self	Willow, Chicory
for others	Centaury, Pine, Red Chestnut, Vervain, Agrimony
PLACID	Oak, Water Violet, Wild Rose, Clematis, Centaury, Mimulus
PLAY-ACT	Chicory, Willow, Vervain, Vine, Clematis
PLEASURE	
none, in life	Mustard, Sweet Chestnut
takes, in company of others	Heather
takes, in converting others	Vervain, Rock Water, Beech
seeks	Agrimony
takes, in being an exhibitionist	Vervain, Vine
PLODDERS	Oak
POISE	
lack of	Scleranthus
possesses	Water Violet
POLLUTION	
sense of being contaminated by	Crab Apple
fear of	Mimulus
agitated by, for fear of harm to others	Red Chestnut
agitated by, on principle	Vervain

Moods	Remedies
PONDER	
on problem-solving	Vervain
on worries/mental arguments	White Chestnut
on future	Clematis
on past	Honeysuckle
on self	Heather, Chicory, Willow
fearfully, about what *might* happen	Aspen
POSSESSIVENESS	Chicory, Heather
POUT	
with resentment	Willow
with self-pity	Chicory, Willow
POWER	
desire for	Vine
desire for, to manipulate	Chicory
frustrated by lack of	Vine, Vervain
PRAGMATIC	Vine, Vervain, Oak, Chicory
PRAISE	
desires	Chicory
seeks, for reassurance	Cerato
wallows in	Vine, Chicory
PREACH	
tendency to	Vervain, Rock Water, Beech
PRECISE	Vervain, Rock Water, Beech

Moods	Remedies
PRE-OCCUPATION	
with thoughts/worries	White Chestnut
with future/fantasy	Clematis
with past	Honeysuckle
with injustice	Vervain
with self	Heather, Rock Water, Crab Apple, Chicory, Willow
with cleanliness	Crab Apple
with detail/trivialities	Crab Apple
with jealousy	Holly, Willow
with grievances	Holly, Willow, Vervain
PRESENTIMENT	Aspen
PRESSURE	
of responsibility, overwhelmed by	Elm
of work, thrives on	Vervain
to serve/assist others	Centaury
unaffected by/takes in stride	Oak
to conform, influenced by	Cerato, Walnut, Centaury
PRESUMPTUOUS	Vine, Chicory, Beech
PRETENCE	
of courage/happiness	Agrimony
PRETENTIOUS	Beech, Chicory, Vine
PRIDE	Water Violet, Rock Water, Chicory, Crab Apple
PRINCIPLES	
feels strongly about	Vervain
PRIVACY	
enjoys, needs	Water Violet

Moods	Remedies
PROCRASTINATION	
through lethargy	Hornbeam
through uncertainty	Scleranthus, Larch
through fear	Mimulus
PROTECTIVE	Centaury, Chicory, Red Chestnut, Vervain, Oak
PROTECTION	
from disturbing outside influences	Walnut
PROUD	Water Violet, Rock Water, Chicory, Crab Apple
PURIST	Rock Water, Vervain, Beech
QUALM	Aspen, Cerato, Pine, Gentian, Rock Water
QUARRELSOME	Willow, Vervain, Holly, Chicory, Beech, Impatiens
QUARRELS	
avoids	Agrimony, Centaury, Clematis, Wild Rose
QUESTIONS	
repeated, for confirmation	Cerato
out of keen interest	Vervain
out of suspicion	Holly, Willow
out of arrogance	Vine, Beech
QUICK	Impatiens, Vervain

Moods	Remedies
QUIET	
generally, by nature	Aspen, Centaury, Scleranthus, Water Violet, Centaury
and dreamy	Clematis
and shy	Mimulus
QUIZZICAL	Cerato, Vervain
RACE AHEAD	
generally disposed to	Impatiens
thoughts tend to	Impatiens, Vervain, White Chestnut, Aspen
RAGE	
uncontrolled/irrational	Cherry Plum
due to authoritarianism	Vine
due to hatred/revenge/envy	Holly
due to injustice/sense of principle	Vervain
due to irritability/impatience	Impatiens
RAPE	
after effects of: shock	Star of Bethlehem, Rescue Remedy
disgust/sense of contamination/ uncleanliness	Crab Apple
guilt	Pine
nightmares/horror	Rock Rose
ghastly memory	Honeysuckle, Rock Rose, Star of Bethlehem
plagued by repetitive thoughts	White Chestnut

Moods	Remedies
RASH	
acts rashly	Impatiens, Vervain
emotionally irritated by physical rash	Impatiens
emotionally feels unclean due to rash	Crab Apple
REACTIVE	
in response to injustice or insult	Vervain
as result of resentment/self pity	Willow, Chicory
as result of humiliation	Vervain, Chicory
as result of humiliation, but absorbed	Water Violet
spitefully or as result of hatred/jealousy	Holly
in authoritarian manner	Vine
in form of rage/uncontrolled temper	Cherry Plum
REALITY	
no sense of/ungrounded	Clematis
firm sense of	Oak, Vervain, Vine
REALIZATION (sudden)	Star of Bethlehem
REASSURANCE	
needs/seeks due to uncertainty	Cerato
needs, to encourage	Mimulus, Larch
REBELLIOUSNESS	Beech, Impatiens, Vervain, Vine
REBIRTHING	
adjustment to/after	Walnut
shock, as result of	Star of Bethlehem
guilt, uncovered by	Pine
grief/sadness, uncovered by	Star of Bethlehem
inability to forgive, uncovered by	Willow
self condemnation/disgust, as result of	Crab Apple

Moods	Remedies
RECEPTIVE	
to other people's needs	Centaury, Walnut, Red Chestnut, Chicory
to fantasies/creativity	Clematis
RECLUSE, by preference	Water Violet
due to fear	Aspen, Mimulus, Rock Rose, Cherry Plum
due to fear of contamination from outside	Crab Apple
as mark of self-martyrdom/ self-perfectionism	Rock Water
due to resentment	Willow
RECOIL	
through shock	Star of Bethlehem
through disgust	Crab Apple
through horror	Rock Rose
through fear	Aspen, Mimulus, Rock Rose
through abusive verbal attack	Walnut, Mimulus, Centaury, Agrimony
RECOVERY	
adjustment during	Walnut
depletion of energy during	Hornbeam, Olive
depressed/weepy during	Mustard, Willow, Gorse (if due to poor prognosis)
diseased feeling during	Crab Apple
shock to the system during	Star of Bethlehem, Rescue Remedy
set-back during	Gentian
despair of serious set-back	Sweet Chestnut
RECTITUDE	Rock Water, Vervain
REFORMER	Rock Water, Vervain

Moods	Remedies
REFRACTORY	Beech, Vine, Vervain, Impatiens
REFUSAL to conform	
due to own strength of character	Beech, Vervain, Vine, Chicory
due to unconventionalist ideas	Clematis
REFUSAL TO BE CONSOLED	
after shocking news	Star of Bethlehem
wishes to be left alone to grieve/	
reflect in peace and silence	Water Violet, Honeysuckle
as shows signs of weakness	Vine, Rock Water
yet manipulates consolation and	
sympathy through self-pity	Chicory, Willow
has innate courage to face	
adversity	Oak
REGARD FOR SELF	
poor, due to self-detestation	Crab Apple
poor, due to guilt/self-reproach	Pine
high, but wants to be better	Rock Water
REGRESSION	
with thoughts of past	Honeysuckle
shocked/saddened by	Star of Bethlehem
frightened by	Mimulus, Rock Rose
adjustment to	Walnut
depressed by/denting ambition	Gentian
REGRETS	Honeysuckle, Pine

Moods	Remedies
REJECTION	
with grief/sense of loss or shock	Star of Bethlehem
with self-blame	Pine, Crab Apple
with resentment/bitterness	Willow
with hatred/jealousy	Holly
with no confidence	Larch
with sense of vulnerability	Cerato, Mimulus, Larch
with over-concern/fearful anxiety over others	Red Chestnut
with over-concern/possessiveness	Chicory, Heather
RELAPSE	
into old unproductive habits	Chestnut Bud
depressed by	Gentian
RELAXATION	
difficult, due to tension	Vervain, Rock Water, Vine
easy, due to drowsiness	Olive, Clematis
easy, due to apathy/lethargy	Wild Rose, Hornbeam
difficult due to worrying thoughts	White Chestnut
difficult due to fear/anxiety	Mimulus, Aspen, Rock Rose, Cherry Plum
difficult due to fear for others	Red Chestnut
difficult due to impatience/cannot slow down	Impatiens, Vervain
see also RESTLESSNESS	
RELEASE	
longs for, from servile work	Centaury
longs for, as escape from present circumstances	Clematis
longs for, from life	Clematis
longs for, from anguish	Sweet Chestnut
longs for, from guilt	Pine
longs for, from torment	Agrimony, White Chestnut
longs for, from contamination of disease	Crab Apple

Moods	Remedies
RELENTLESS	Oak, Vervain
REMINDED	
and saddened by memories	Honeysuckle
needs to be, due to forgetfulness	Clematis
needs to be, due to full mind	White Chestnut, Vervain
needs to be, repeatedly	Chestnut Bud, Clematis
irritated at being reminded of short-comings	Vervain, Vine, Impatiens
REMINDERS	
nostalgic	Honeysuckle
sentimental	Walnut, Honeysuckle
which provoke guilt	Pine
which provoke sadness/grief	Star of Bethlehem, Honeysuckle
which provoke self disgust	Crab Apple
about injustice	Vervain
which revive grudges	Willow
which cause set-back	Gentian
REMINISCENCE	Honeysuckle
REMORSE	Pine
REMOTENESS	
due to mental escapism/ day-dreaming	Clematis
due to absorption with past	Honeysuckle
due to grief/shock	Star of Bethlehem
due to utter dejection/emptiness	Sweet Chestnut
through desire for private solitude	Water Violet
suffered by sensitive people	Larch, Mimulus, Centaury, Crab Apple
RENUNCIATION	Rock Water

Moods	Remedies
REPEAT	
same mistakes	Chestnut Bud
oneself verbally	Heather, Vervain, Impatiens
REPELLED	Crab Apple
REPENTING	Pine
REPRESSED EMOTIONS	
generally	Agrimony, Centaury, Water Violet
of guilt	Pine
of indecision	Scleranthus
of resentment/bitterness	Willow
festering thoughts/mental arguments	White Chestnut
REPUGNANCE	Crab Apple
REPULSION	
generally	Crab Apple
through horror	Star of Bethlehem, Rock Rose
RESENTMENT	Willow
vengeful	Holly
due to injustice	Vervain
when unappreciated	Chicory, Willow
due to jealousy/envy	Holly
RESERVED	
shy	Mimulus
subservient/weak	Centaury
by choice due to private nature	Water Violet
RESIGNATION	Wild Rose, Gorse
RESILIENCE	Oak, Vervain, Rock Water

Moods	Remedies
RESPECT	
demands	Vine
yearns for, selfishly	Chicory
appreciates	Vervain
deserving of	Water Violet
RESPONSIBILITY	
capable and thrives on	Vervain
copes unflustered with	Oak
feels overwhelmed by	Elm
despondency due to	Elm, Gentian
lost confidence due to	Elm, Larch
carries it with quiet dignified pride	Water Violet
RESTLESSNESS	
through mental torture/worries	Agrimony, White Chestnut
through indecision	Scleranthus
through impatience	Impatiens
through over-enthusiasm	Vervain
through apprehensive anxiety/fears	Aspen, Mimulus, Red Chestnut
see also RELAXATION	
RESTRAINT	
self-inflicted	Rock Water
RETICENCE	
due to indecision	Scleranthus, Cerato
due to doubt	Cerato, Gentian
due to fear/apprehension	Mimulus, Aspen
due to lack of confidence	Larch, Cerato
due to suspicion	Holly

Moods	Remedies
RETIREMENT	
adjustment to/feels unsettled by	Walnut
finds it hard to "switch off" from active work	Vervain
causing recoil due to unaccustomed inactivity	Vervain, Willow, Clematis, Honeysuckle
causing uncertainty about future/ feels lost	Wild Oat
RETROSPECTION	Honeysuckle, Pine, Gorse, Willow
REVENGE	Holly
REVOLT	
at uncleanliness	Crab Apple
at injustice/unfairness	Vervain, Willow
at restrictions/slowness	Impatiens, Vervain, Vine
RIDICULE	
affected by	Mimulus, Centaury, Cerato, Scleranthus, Larch
despondency due to	Gentian
protection from influence of	Walnut
spitefully inflicting	Holly
arrogantly inflicting	Beech, Vine
RIGHT	
arrogantly believes one is always	Vine
believes one's principles are	Vervain, Beech, Rock Water
uncertain that one is	Cerato
RIGHTEOUS	Rock Water, Beech, Vervain
RIGIDITY, mental	Rock Water, Beech, Vine, Vervain

Moods	Remedies
ROCK-SOLID	
and dependable	Oak
and convincingly determined	Vine
ROMANTIC	Clematis
RULE	
desire to	Vine
RULED	
through lack of inner strength	Centaury, Agrimony
due to susceptibility to influence	Cerato, Walnut
rebels against attempts to be	Vine, Vervain, Beech
RUNS AWAY FROM	
responsibility	Elm
problems	Agrimony, Clematis
RUSHED	
sense of being	Impatiens
hyperactivity	Vervain, Impatiens
RUT	
sense of being in	Wild Rose, Clematis, Gorse
RUTHLESSNESS	Vine
SACRIFICE	
self	Rock Water, Pine, Crab Apple, Red Chestnut
self, as martyr	Rock Water, Chicory
SADNESS	Star of Bethlehem, Pine, Sweet Chestnut, Mustard, Willow

Moods	Remedies
SADISTIC	
spiteful/hateful	Holly
and vindictive, with desire to control	Vine
SAFETY	
fear for others	Red Chestnut
fear for one's own	Mimulus, Rescue Remedy
SANCTIMONIOUS	Rock Water, Beech, Vervain, Vine
SANITY	
fear for one's own	Cherry Plum
SARCASTIC	Holly, Willow, Vine, Beech, Chicory
SARDONIC	Willow, Holly, Beech, Vine
SATISFACTION	
lack of, with ambitions	Wild Oat
lack of, with life	Wild Rose, Hornbeam, Gorse, Sweet Chestnut
lack of, with self	Rock Water, Cerato, Crab Apple
SCARED	
generally	Rock Rose, Mimulus, Aspen
for others	Red Chestnut
without knowing why	Aspen
for sanity	Cherry Plum
SCATHING	Holly, Beech
SCATTER-BRAINED	Clematis, Scleranthus, Cherry Plum

Moods	Remedies
SCEPTICAL	Beech, Vine, Gorse, Holly
SCRUFFINESS	
cannot tolerate	Rock Water, Crab Apple
prefers	Wild Rose, Hornbeam, Gorse
SECRETIVE	
out of suspicion for others' motives	Holly
for power/self importance	Vine
enjoys being/clings selfishly to secrets/uses as way of manipulating attention	Chicory
due to desire for privacy	Water Violet
due to fear	Mimulus, Aspen, Rock Rose
due to denial	Agrimony
due to indecision	Scleranthus
due to shame	Crab Apple, Pine
with torturous thoughts	White Chestnut, Agrimony
SECURITY (emotional)	
seeks	Cerato, Mimulus, Heather, Chicory
SEDATE	
due to listlessness	Wild Rose, Hornbeam
due to drowsiness	Clematis, Olive, Hornbeam
composed/clean living/private person	Water Violet
SELF-ABSORPTION	Heather, Willow, Chicory, Rock Water, Beech, Crab Apple

Moods	Remedies
SELF-ABUSE	Crab Apple
SELF-BLAME	Pine
SELF-CENTRED	Chicory, Heather, Willow

SELF-CONFIDENCE

lack of	Larch
lack of, through fear	Mimulus
lack of, momentarily, when under pressure	Elm
lack of, through self distrust	Cerato
lack of, through indecision	Scleranthus
lack of, through feeling of hopelessness	Gorse

SELF-CONSCIOUSNESS	Mimulus, Larch, Cherry Plum

SELF-CONTROL

possesses, by nature	Water Violet, Oak
lack of	Cherry Plum, Holly
may lose, when seriously provoked	Vervain

SELF-DENIAL

inclined to, by nature	Centaury, Rock Water, Red Chestnut, Pine
in a selfish manner – "don't worry about me"	Chicory

SELF-DETERMINATION	Vervain, Oak, Rock Water, Vine
SELF-DISLIKE	Crab Apple
SELF-DISTRUST	Cerato

SELF-ESTEEM

lack of	Larch, Cerato, Pine, Crab Apple, Elm

Moods	Remedies
SELF-IMPORTANT	Chicory, Heather, Vine
SELF-INDULGENT	Chicory, Heather
then feels disgusted	Crab Apple
then feels guilty	Pine
SELF-INTEREST	Chicory, Heather, Rock Water, Beech, Willow
SELF-MARTYRDOM	Centaury, Rock Water, Chicory, Willow
SELF-OPINIONATED	Vine, Vervain, Beech, Chicory
SELF-PITY	Willow, Chicory
SELF-RELIANT	Impatiens, Vine, Water Violet, Oak, Vervain
SELF-REPROACH	Pine
SELF-RESPECT	
lack of	Pine, Crab Apple, Cerato
SELF-RIGHTEOUS	Rock Water, Beech, Vervain
SELF-SACRIFICIAL	
by nature	Rock Water
to gain sympathy	Chicory, Willow
SELF-SUFFICIENT	Water Violet, Oak, Vine
SELFISH	Chicory

Moods	Remedies
SENSITIVITY	
to noise	Clematis, Mimulus, Water Violet, Impatiens
to controversy/conflict/strife	Agrimony, Mimulus, Centaury
sensitive by nature	Walnut, Centaury, Agrimony, Clematis
to criticism	Willow, Chicory, Vervain

see also CRIES EASILY, TEARFULNESS and WEEPINESS

Moods	Remedies
SENTIMENTAL	Honeysuckle, Walnut, Chicory, Red Chestnut, Centaury, Pine
SERENITY	Water Violet
SERVICE	
enjoys giving	Oak, Centaury, Chicory, Red Chestnut, Agrimony
begrudges giving	Willow
SERVILE	Centaury, Agrimony, Pine
SET-BACKS	
discouraged by	Gentian
perseveres in spite of	Oak
gives in to	Gorse
frightened by	Mimulus
SEVERE	Vine, Rock Water

Moods	Remedies
SEX	
dislike of	Crab Apple
afraid of	Mimulus, Larch
feels interfered by	Water Violet
over-excited about	Vervain, Impatiens
dominant	Vine
disinterested in	Clematis, Olive, Hornbeam, Wild Rose
SHAME	Crab Apple, Pine
SHATTERED	
by news	Star of Bethlehem, Rescue Remedy
by exhaustion	Olive
by over-work	Vervain, Oak, Centaury
by stress	Vervain, Elm, Agrimony
in crisis situation	Rescue Remedy
SHOCK	Star of Bethlehem, Rescue Remedy
SHOW-OFF	
knows everything – big "I am"	Vine
due to insecurity	Agrimony
due to excitement/enthusiasm	Vervain
to attract attention	Chicory, Heather
SHRUG	
with resignation/apathy	Wild Rose
with disinterest	Clematis, Hornbeam, Olive
with despondency	Gentian, Gorse
with self-pity	Willow
with indignation	Chicory
SHYNESS	Mimulus

Moods	Remedies
SICKNESS	
generally	Crab Apple
through travel	Scleranthus
see also ILLNESS and AILMENTS	
SILENCE	
enjoys	Water Violet, Clematis
SIN	
believes one has committed	Pine
SINCERE	Vervain, Oak, Water Violet, Red Chestnut, Centaury
SKITTISH	Impatiens, Scleranthus, Mimulus, Aspen
SLEEP	
easily	Clematis
unrefreshingly	Hornbeam, Wild Rose
desires, due to exhaustion	Olive
SLEEPLESSNESS	
through worry/mental arguments/ tormented thoughts	White Chestnut
through tension	Vervain, Rock Water
through over-exhaustion	Olive
through grief	Star of Bethlehem, Honeysuckle, Rescue Remedy
through restlessness	Vervain, Agrimony, Impatiens
through anxiety	Aspen, Agrimony
through fear	Mimulus, Rock Rose

Moods	Remedies
SLOW	
in learning/correcting past mistakes	Chestnut Bud
because of lack of interest	Clematis
because of indecision	Scleranthus
to get started	Hornbeam
SLOWNESS	
irritated by	Impatiens
SMILE	
covers feelings	Agrimony
finds it hard to (depressed)	Mustard, Willow, Gorse, Sweet Chestnut
SMOTHER	
with love	Chicory
SMUG	Vine, Chicory, Holly, Rock Water, Beech
SNOOTY	Vine, Rock Water, Water Violet, Beech
SNOBBISHNESS	Rock Water, Beech, Vine, Heather, Chicory
SOCIABLE	Agrimony, Vervain, Chicory, Heather
SOLACE	
needs after bad news/shock	Star of Bethlehem
needs after disappointment	Gentian
desire for quietude	Water Violet
wants to be left alone to brood	Willow

Moods	Remedies
SOLITARY	
by choice, preference for privacy	Water Violet
by choice, to work at own pace	Impatiens
strong aversion to being	Heather
by choice, for escapism	Clematis
SORROWFUL	
due to grief/loss	Star of Bethlehem
utterly forlorn/dejected	Sweet Chestnut
due to self-pity	Willow, Chicory
for unknown reason	Mustard
remembering past/good old days	Honeysuckle
easily affected by sentiment	Honeysuckle, Walnut, Red Chestnut, Chicory
SORRY	Pine
SPACED OUT	Clematis
SPELL-BOUND	Clematis, Centaury
SPIRITLESS	
due to depression	Mustard, Gorse, Sweet Chestnut
due to self-pity	Willow
due to apathy	Wild Rose
due to disinterest	Clematis, Honeysuckle
due to deep sadness	Star of Bethlehem, Sweet Chestnut
due to lost direction	Wild Oat, Walnut
due to subservience	Centaury
due to fear	Mimulus, Larch
SPIRITUALITY	
to regain sense of	Walnut, Clematis, Willow, Holly, Wild Oat
SPITEFULNESS	Holly, Chicory

Moods	Remedies
SPOOKED	Star of Bethlehem, Aspen, Rock Rose, Rescue Remedy
SQUEAMISHNESS	Mimulus, Crab Apple
STAGE-FRIGHT	
panic due to	Rock Rose, Cherry Plum, Rescue Remedy
worry prior to	White Chestnut, Aspen, Mimulus
due to lack of confidence	Larch
hides behind exuberance	Agrimony
STAGNATION	
due to listlessness	Wild Rose
due to disinterest	Honeysuckle, Gorse, Mustard, Willow
due to despondency	Gentian
due to inability to learn from experience	Chestnut Bud
help to move on	Walnut (in addition to remedy for cause)
STAMINA	
possesses	Oak, Vervain, Vine, Heather
lack of	Centaury, Gorse, Gentian, Olive, Hornbeam, Clematis, Wild Rose
STAND-OFFISH	
due to private nature (not rudely)	Water Violet
due to suspicion	Holly
due to fear	Mimulus
STARCHY	Rock Water
STARTLED	Star of Bethlehem, Rescue Remedy

Moods	Remedies
STEADFAST	Oak, Vervain, Vine, Water Violet, Chicory
STIGMA	
shame due to	Crab Apple
frustrated/angry about injustice of	Vervain
STOICISM	Water Violet
STRAIN	Impatiens, Rock Water, Vervain
STRANGE SENSATION	
unexplained apprehension	Aspen
unexplained depression	Mustard
as though on a knife edge	Aspen, Impatiens, Vervain
STRANGERS	
frightened of	Mimulus
suspicious of	Holly
searches out	Heather
STRENGTH	
of character	Vine, Vervain, Oak, Water Violet
self-disciplined	Rock Water, Water Violet
in matters of principle	Vervain
in illness/maintains against adversity	Oak
STRICT	
with others	Beech, Chicory, Vervain, Vine
with self	Rock Water
STRIVE	Oak, Vervain

Moods	Remedies
STRUGGLES	
on in spite of adversity	Oak
to make point understood	Vervain
to please others	Centaury
to please self	Rock Water, Pine, Crab Apple
STUBBORNNESS	
generally, by nature	Vervain, Vine, Chicory, Beech
about self-discipline	Rock Water
due to genuine courage	Oak
STUNNED	Star of Bethlehem, Clematis
STUPIDITY	
intolerant of	Beech, Vine, Impatiens
SUBMISSIVE	Centaury
SUBSERVIENT	Centaury
SUCCESS	
fear of	Larch
pessimistic about	Gentian, Larch, Gorse
SUDDEN	
terror/panic	Rock Rose, Rescue Remedy
alarm	Star of Bethlehem
depression/dark cloud descending	Mustard
confrontation, causing fear	Mimulus, Rescue Remedy
SUFFERENCE	
willingly, as martyr	Rock Water, Chicory
endures without complaint	Oak, Centaury, Agrimony
works under, complaining	Willow

Moods	Remedies
SUFFOCATION, emotional	
by possessive love	Chicory
SUICIDE	
irrational desire to commit	Cherry Plum
considers, to escape from fear	Aspen, Agrimony, Rock Rose, Mimulus
fear of committing	Cherry Plum
rationally considers, to escape boredom	Clematis
rationally considers, to escape deep depression	Sweet Chestnut, Gorse, Mustard
rationally considers, to join loved one	Clematis, Honeysuckle
rationally considers, for self-reproach	Pine
considered due to being over-burdened by responsibility or pressures	Elm, Larch, Centaury

NB: White Chestnut in addition to the above is recommended.

SULKINESS	Willow, Chicory
SULLEN	Willow, Gorse
SUPERCILIOUS	Water Violet, Vine, Beech, Rock Water
SUPERFICIAL	Agrimony
SUPERIORITY COMPLEX	Water Violet, Vine, Beech, Rock Water

Moods	Remedies
SUPERNATURAL	
defined fear of	Mimulus, Rock Rose
undefined fear of	Aspen
uncontrolled fear of	Cherry Plum, Rock Rose
feels strong but unwanted influence of	Walnut
seeks companionship with	Clematis
SUPERSTITIOUS	
generally	Rock Water, Mimulus, Rock Rose
influenced by superstition	Walnut
SUPPRESSED EMOTION	
due to shock	Star of Bethlehem
hidden behind cheerfulness	Agrimony
SURE OF THEMSELVES	Vine, Water Violet, Oak, Rock Water
SUSPICION	Holly
SYMPATHY	
wish for	Chicory, Heather, Willow
lack of, for others	Beech, Vine, Holly
SYMPTOMS	
obsessed with detail of	Crab Apple, White Chestnut
obsessed with consequences of	Heather, Mimulus, White Chestnut
unspoken fear of	Agrimony, Mimulus, Aspen, White Chestnut
TACTLESSNESS	Vine, Chicory, Impatiens, Beech, Vervain

Moods	Remedies
TALKATIVE	
generally	Heather, Chicory, Cerato, Vervain, Agrimony
about self	Heather
for attention	Heather, Chicory
for reassurance/guidance	Cerato
about the past	Honeysuckle
with explanations, opinions	Vervain
nervously, about fears	Rock Rose, Mimulus, Cherry Plum
nervously, as means of masking troubles	Agrimony
impatiently	Impatiens
TALKS QUICKLY	
by nature	Impatiens, Heather
because of fear/anxiety	Agrimony, Mimulus, Impatiens
due to over-enthusiasm	Vervain
TANTRUMS	Cherry Plum, Holly, Impatiens, Vervain
to ease transition in childhood	Walnut
TEARFULNESS	
easily prone to, out of self pity	Chicory, Willow
through instability	Scleranthus
through despair	Sweet Chestnut
through utter exhaustion	Olive
due to sensitivity	Centaury, Mimulus, Red Chestnut, Walnut
easily moved, due to sensitivity to influence	Walnut
through sentimentality	Honeysuckle, Walnut
hidden/cries alone	Water Violet, Agrimony

see also CRIES EASILY, SENSITIVITY and WEEPINESS

Moods	Remedies
TEDIUM	
life/work etc., seems full of	Clematis, Hornbeam, Wild Rose
irritated by	Impatiens, Vervain, Vine, Beech
TEMPER	
violent, uncontrolled	Cherry Plum
quick, fiery	Impatiens, Vervain, Vine, Holly
unstable	Scleranthus, Cherry Plum
controlled, but frustrated annoyance due to restriction or incapacity	Oak
TEMPTATION	
influenced by	Cerato, Walnut, Centaury
influenced by, due to greed	Chicory
TENSION	
suffers by nature	Beech, Impatiens, Rock Water, Vervain, Vine
due to shock	Star of Bethlehem
through fear	Mimulus, Aspen, Rock Rose, Cherry Plum
through fear for others	Red Chestnut
through concerned fretfulness over others	Chicory, Red Chestnut
TENTATIVE	Mimulus, Larch, Cerato, Scleranthus
TERROR	Rock Rose
TERSE	Impatiens, Vine
TETCHY	Impatiens, Beech, Willow

Moods	Remedies
THANKS	
expects, desires	Chicory
THEATRICAL	
to hide feelings/make light of situation	Agrimony
self-indulgent/attention seeking	Chicory, Heather, Willow
over-enthusiastic/uncontrollably	Vervain, Cherry Plum
due to jealousy/envy of others' success	Holly
due to panic (see *also* STAGE FRIGHT)	Rescue Remedy
THICK-SKINNED	Vine
THOUGHTS	
persistent, worrying	White Chestnut
of future	Clematis
of past	Honeysuckle
of revenge	Holly, Willow
unrealistic/irrational dread	Cherry Plum, Aspen
miserable	Willow, Gorse
frustrated	Agrimony, Walnut, Vervain
THOUGHTFUL	
over (lost in thought/dreamy)	Clematis
THWARTED	
frustrated	Vervain, Impatiens, Beech, Walnut
feels hurt when	Chicory
TIME	
careless with/no sense of	Clematis, Wild Rose
impatient with	Impatiens
over-concerned with	Impatiens, Vervain, Rock Water, Beech

Moods	Remedies
TIMIDITY	Mimulus, Centaury, Larch

TIRED

generally	Olive, Hornbeam
sleepy drowsy/escapist	Clematis
with life	Sweet Chestnut

NB: Important to acknowledge and treat cause

TIRESOME

due to negative outlook	Willow
due to nagging	Chicory
due to talkativeness	Heather
due to apathetic lack of interest	Wild Rose
of others if not listening, taking no notice, not obeying, being too slow or stupid	Vervain, Vine, Impatiens, Beech

TIRELESS	Oak, Vervain, Rock Water, Vine

TOLERANCE

lack of	Beech, Chicory, Vine, Vervain, Impatiens

TOMORROW

looking forward to	Clematis
afraid of	Mimulus, Aspen
worried about	White Chestnut
cannot wait to arrive	Impatiens

TONGUE-TIED

through shyness/lack of confidence/ self-consciousness	Mimulus, Larch
through impatience/trying to talk too quickly	Impatiens, Vervain

Moods	Remedies
TORMENTED	
by hidden worries	Agrimony
by persistent thoughts	White Chestnut
by fears	Aspen, Rock Rose, Mimulus, Red Chestnut
by anguish	Sweet Chestnut
by thoughts of jealousy/envy	Holly
by fear of losing control	Cherry Plum
TOTALITARIAN	Vine
TOUGH	Vine, Vervain, Oak, Chicory
TOXICITY	
feeling of contamination by	Crab Apple
TRANQUILLITY	
enjoys/needs, by nature	Water Violet, Clematis, Wild Rose, Mimulus, Centaury
seeks, due to sensitivity	Walnut
seeks, due to troubled thoughts	White Chestnut, Agrimony, Scleranthus
seeks, due to fear of others and forced situations	Mimulus, Larch
TRANSFIXED	
in deep thought/bemused	Clematis
after shock	Star of Bethlehem, Rescue Remedy
TRANSITION	Walnut
TRAUMA	Star of Bethlehem, Rescue Remedy
TRAVEL-SICK	Rescue Remedy, Scleranthus

Moods	Remedies
TREMBLE	
for no reason	Aspen
with fear	Mimulus, Aspen, Rock Rose
with effects of shock	Star of Bethlehem
TRENCHANT	Vervain, Impatiens, Vine
TRIP (hallucinatory)	
frightened by	Rock Rose, Aspen, Mimulus, Rescue Remedy
disturbed by	Honeysuckle, Walnut
shocked by	Star of Bethlehem
bemused by	Clematis
flashbacks after	Honeysuckle, Walnut
TRIVIALITIES	
obsessed with	Crab Apple, Impatiens, Beech
TRUST	
lack of, in others	Holly
lack of, in self	Cerato
TRUTH	
seeking	Wild Oat, Vervain
TRUTHFULNESS	
concerned for	Vervain
TURBULENT THOUGHTS	Agrimony, White Chestnut
TURMOIL, mental	Agrimony, White Chestnut, Scleranthus
TYRANNICAL	Vine

Moods	Remedies
UBIQUITOUS	Vervain
UGLY	
believes one is	Crab Apple
ULTERIOR MOTIVE	
to control	Vine, Chicory
to possess	Chicory
for vengeance	Holly
for sympathy	Willow, Chicory
UMBRAGE	Chicory, Willow
UNASSUMING	Mimulus, Centaury, Clematis, Wild Rose, Larch
UNAWARE	Clematis, Wild Rose
UNCERTAINTY	Scleranthus
through self-distrust	Cerato
through lack of faith	Gentian, Cerato
through lack of hope	Gorse
through lack of strength	Hornbeam
of ambitions	Wild Oat
due to doubt of ability to cope with responsibility	Elm
due to lack of confidence	Larch
UNCLEANLINESS, feeling of	Crab Apple
UNCOMPLAINING	
through resignation	Wild Rose
through disinterest	Clematis
courage	Oak
pretended courage	Agrimony
UNCONVENTIONAL	
due to creative, futuristic tendencies	Wild Oat, Clematis
to create own standards	Vine

Moods	Remedies
UNDERSTANDING	
lack of	Beech, Vine, Impatiens
at times, when against own standards	Chicory, Vervain
UNEASINESS	
vague sense of apprehensive	Aspen
in company of others	Mimulus, Larch
UNGROUNDED	Clematis
UNHAPPY	
with present	Clematis
for no reason	Mustard
due to bitterness/self pity	Willow
due to jealousy	Holly
due to longing for past	Honeysuckle
due to guilt	Pine
due to exhaustion	Olive
with self	Scleranthus, Cerato, Crab Apple, Pine, Rock Water, Larch, Centaury
UNKNOWN CAUSES	
of depression	Mustard
of fear	Aspen
UNNERVED	Mimulus, Walnut, Aspen
UNOBSERVANT	Clematis
UNPREDICTABLE	Scleranthus, Cherry Plum, Clematis, Impatiens
UNREASONABLE	
with others	Vine, Beech, Impatiens
with self	Rock Water

Moods	Remedies
UNRELIABLE	
because of uncertainty	Scleranthus
because of self-distrust	Cerato
because easily influenced	Centaury, Cerato, Agrimony, Mimulus
UNREST	
due to tension	Vervain
due to mental arguments/worry	White Chestnut, Agrimony
due to fear	Mimulus, Aspen, Rock Rose, Red Chestnut
due to agitation/irritability	Impatiens, Beech, Vervain
due to inner torment	Agrimony
due to vexatious thoughts	Holly
due to fear of losing control	Cherry Plum
due to violent imaginings	Cherry Plum
due to indecision	Scleranthus
UPTIGHT	Vervain, Impatiens, Rock Water, Beech, Vine
UNSETTLED	
generally	Walnut
by worry	White Chestnut
by indecision	Scleranthus
by guilt	Pine
USED	
feels used by others	Centaury, Chicory, Willow
USELESSNESS, sense of	Cerato, Pine, Gentian, Gorse, Larch, Elm
VACANT EXPRESSION	Clematis, Wild Rose

Moods	Remedies
VAGUE	Clematis, Cerato, Scleranthus, Wild Rose
VAIN	Beech, Rock Water, Chicory, Heather
VARIABLE MOOD	Scleranthus, Mustard, Cerato, Walnut
VEHEMENCE	Vervain, Impatiens, Cherry Plum, Holly, Beech
VEIL	
cast for privacy	Water Violet
cast as means of hiding feelings	Agrimony
VENGEFUL	
through hate/spite/revenge	Holly
fear of being	Cherry Plum
VENOMOUS	Holly
VERBOSE	Heather, Vervain
VERVE	Vervain
VEXED	Impatiens, Beech, Holly, Vervain
VICTIMISED	Centaury, Mimulus
feels, and resents being	Willow, Chicory
irrationally fears one is being	Cherry Plum, Holly
VINDICTIVE	Holly, Chicory
VIOLENT	
rage	Cherry Plum
fear of being	Cherry Plum
satisfaction from being/desire to be	Holly
to show superiority	Vine

Moods	Remedies
VITALITY	
sapped by others	Agrimony, Centaury, Clematis, Mimulus, Larch
saps others	Cerato, Chicory, Heather
drained of/exhausted	Hornbeam, Olive
VIVACIOUS	Agrimony, Impatiens, Vervain
VOCAL	
at any opportunity, about self	Heather
opinionated about beliefs	Vervain
self-opinionated	Vine
VOCATION	
uncertain of	Wild Oat, Cerato
VOLATILE	Scleranthus, Mustard, Holly
VOMIT	
fear of	Mimulus, Crab Apple
disgust of	Crab Apple
VOO-DOO	
vague apprehension about	Aspen
terrified of	Rock Rose
influenced by	Walnut
desire to rid oneself of	Crab Apple, Walnut
VULNERABILITY	Centaury, Scleranthus, Walnut, Mimulus, Larch, Chestnut Bud, Cerato
WAIL	
for attention	Chicory, Willow
with utter despair	Sweet Chestnut
with feelings of remorse	Pine

Moods	Remedies
WALLOW	
in self pity	Willow, Chicory
see also MARTYR	
WANDER AIMLESSLY in life	
by nature, due to apathy	Wild Rose
due to unfulfilled ambitions	Wild Oat
due to lack of interest	Clematis
due to disappointing set-backs/ hopelessness	Gentian, Gorse
WARY	
through suspicion	Holly
through fear	Mimulus
through reasonable caution	Oak, Vervain, Water Violet
WEAKNESS	
doubt of mental strength	Hornbeam
weak-willed	Centaury
exhausted	Olive
WEAK-WILLED	
by nature	Centaury
through shyness/timidity	Mimulus
through lack of confidence	Larch
WEARINESS	
through exhaustion	Olive
through listlessness	Hornbeam, Wild Rose
from over-work, but keeps going	Centaury, Oak, Rock Water
WEEP	
easily	Chicory, Heather, Willow
unable to, due to numbness (e.g. following serious news)	Star of Bethlehem, Agrimony, Walnut
unable to, due to self-denial	Rock Water

Moods	Remedies
WEEPINESS	
out of self-pity	Chicory, Willow, Heather
with utter despair	Sweet Chestnut
with remorse	Pine
with grief	Star of Bethlehem, Sweet Chestnut, Honeysuckle
with sentimentality	Walnut, Honeysuckle
with relief	Agrimony
weeps alone/hides tears from others	Water Violet, Agrimony

see also CRIES EASILY, SENSITIVITY and TEARFULNESS

WEIRD FEELINGS	Cherry Plum, Clematis
WICKEDNESS	Holly
fear of acting in	Cherry Plum
WILD	Cherry Plum
WILL	
strong	Beech, Chicory, Rock Water, Vervain, Vine
weak	Centaury
weak on occasions	Agrimony, Walnut
strength of character	Oak
WISDOM	
lacks	Chestnut Bud, Cerato
WISE	Water Violet, Oak, Vervain
WISHFUL	Clematis, Honeysuckle
with regrets	Pine, Honeysuckle
WISTFUL	Clematis, Honeysuckle

Moods	Remedies
WITHDRAWAL	
from drugs/alcohol/tobacco etc.,	
– helps adjustment during	Walnut
– helps learn from experience	Chestnut Bud
– helps to cleanse mind/body	Crab Apple
– helps strengthen will to resist	Hornbeam, Centaury

*NB: Important to treat underlying cause of addiction
see also ADDICTION*

WITHDRAWN	
from society through shyness	Mimulus
due to desire for privacy	Water Violet
by hiding from/ignoring existence	
of problems	Agrimony
sulkily, due to self-pity	Willow
due to distrust/suspicion	Holly
as means of escape	Clematis
due to pre-occupation with worry	White Chestnut
having lost all hope	Gorse, Sweet Chestnut

WONDERS	
about future event	Clematis

WORKAHOLIC	
by nature	Vervain, Oak, Rock Water
servile	Centaury

WORRY	
generally	White Chestnut
over other people's troubles	Red Chestnut
over own troubles	Heather
hidden	Agrimony
fussily	Chicory, Vervain
with mental arguments	White Chestnut
welfare of others	Vervain, Red Chestnut, Chicory

WORTHINESS	
low sense of	Pine, Crab Apple, Larch

Moods	Remedies
WRONG-DOING	
blames self/feels guilty, for others' mistakes	Pine
blames others	Willow, Beech, Vine, Chicory
condemns self for	Crab Apple, Pine, Rock Water
X-RAY	
feels contaminated by	Crab Apple
feels need for protection from	Walnut, Crab Apple
fear of	Mimulus, Rock Rose
persistent worry over	White Chestnut, Crab Apple
"YES"	
"yes person", cannot say "no"	Centaury
agrees against own natural instincts	Mimulus, Larch, Centaury, Cerato, Walnut
YEARNING	
for better times	Clematis
for past	Honeysuckle
for youth	Honeysuckle
for love	Chicory
for loved ones	Red Chestnut, Chicory
covetously/for selfish reasons	Chicory, Holly
YOGA	
to calm mind of worry, prior to	White Chestnut, Agrimony, Walnut
to relax mind of tension, prior to	Vervain, Rock Water, Beech, Holly

Moods	Remedies
YOUTHFULNESS	
obsessive preservation of	Rock Water, Crab Apple, Heather, Honeysuckle
obsessed with, due to fear of ageing	Rock Rose, Mimulus, Agrimony
obsessed with physical state/pushes self to over-exercise/stay fit	Rock Water
ZEALOUS	Vervain
ZEST	
lack of, through exhaustion	Olive
lack of, through listlessness	Hornbeam, Wild Rose
lack of, through disinterest	Clematis, Wild Rose, Mustard
lack of, through depression	Mustard, Sweet Chestnut, Gorse, Gentian, Willow
lack of, through worry	White Chestnut
ZOMBIE-LIKE	
as in dream state	Clematis
apathetic/blank	Wild Rose
through depression	Mustard, Gorse, Sweet Chestnut
through exhaustion	Olive
mentally stunned, through shock	Star of Bethlehem, Rescue Remedy

USEFUL ADDRESSES

The Dr. Edward Bach Centre/The Dr. Edward Bach Foundation
Mount Vernon,
Sotwell, Wallingford,
Oxon. OX10 0PZ
United Kingdom
(advice and information about Bach Flower Remedies, education, training and registration of counsellors in the Bach Flower Remedies)

Bach Flower Remedies Ltd.,
Broadheath House,
83 Parkside,
Wimbledon,
London SW19 5LP
United Kingdom
(local stockists, worldwide distribution and all overseas enquiries)

Nelsons Homoeopathic Pharmacy
73 Duke Street,
London W1M 6BY
United Kingdom
(Nelson homoeopathic and Bach Flower Remedy UK mail order)